LIFE, DEATH AND AID

LIFE, DEATH AND AID

The *Médecins Sans Frontières* Report on World Crisis Intervention

Edited by François Jean

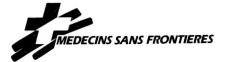

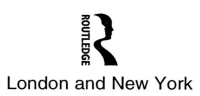

London and New York

English language edition first published 1993
by Routledge
11 New Fetter Lane, London EC4P 4EE

Simultaneously published in the USA and Canada
by Routledge
29 West 35th Street, New York, NY 10001

Typeset in Garamond by LaserScript, Mitcham, Surrey
Printed and bound in Great Britain by
Biddles Ltd, Guildford and King's Lynn

British Library Cataloguing in Publication Data
A catalogue record for this book is available from the British Library.

Library of Congress Cataloging in Publication Data
Has been applied for

ISBN 0–415–10550–1

CONTENTS

CONTENTS

'Humanitarian' military intervention

FOREWORD

Every November on its International Day for Populations in Danger, Médecins Sans Frontières tries to draw the attention of public opinion to the ten most urgent humanitarian crises in the world. Over the past two years, the sweeping pace of change in world crisis intervention – be it in Somalia, the former Yugoslavia or Liberia – has been so overwhelming that MSF, as a non-governmental humanitarian organization, has had to take time to sit back and reflect on a heavily publicized, albeit hazy, concept: the response of the international community to crisis.

Since the Cold War ground to a halt, the international order has altered sharply and the nature of crisis intervention has had to change accordingly. New theories are abounding, new mechanisms have been created and new participants are appearing on an increasingly complex humanitarian scene. More importantly, humanitarian aid is increasingly being brought under governmental control – thus taking on a military aspect – while the task of guaranteeing humanitarian relief and world peace is being left up to the United Nations.

Three great changes have taken place, all of which have had an effect on the crises themselves, the international reactions they have provoked and the role of the media. The most worrying trend to affect humanitarian aid is that relief operations are now being launched in increasingly volatile and fragmented troublespots, where it can be hard to differentiate between the supposed rulers and the gang leaders.

Aid agencies are now finding it more difficult to reach victims, as security conditions have become precarious and warring parties are clearly showing a diminishing respect for humanitarian organizations. The growing links between aid and politics are accentuating this situation. In Somalia and Yugoslavia, for example, the neutrality, impartiality and independence of aid operations, essential conditions for intervention, are being put into question – with some justification – by the very recipients of aid.

The main root of the problem lies with states becoming more directly involved in humanitarian aid. During the last century or, to be more precise, since the creation of the concept of humanitarian aid by Henri Dunant, the founder of the Red Cross, volunteers have followed armies on to the battlefield to care for war victims. Now it is the armies themselves that 'accompany' humanitarian organizations to the front line. This new military involvement in relief work has opened a Pandora's box: the motivations, methods and objectives of humanitarian aid have been turned upside down. As a result, humanitarian organizations are protesting their impartiality while rethinking their collaboration with the United Nations and individual governments.

Finally, the media have never played such an ambiguous role in humanitarian relief. Live TV coverage, as opposed to real needs, is now dictating the priorities of humanitarian operations. Prime time footage of the UN's 'humanitarian' intervention on Mogadishu beach allowed television cameras to gloss over the traps inherent in the hope-restoring operation. Similarly, the highly publicized rescue of Sarajevo's little Irma, while fooling no one about its public relations value, managed temporarily to obscure the realities of the relief situation in the former Yugoslavia while forcing the United Nations to bend their criteria on medical evacuations.

Life, Death and Aid focuses on the most critical situations of the day, each chosen primarily on the basis of conflict or internal strife, forced movements of populations and, sometimes, famines and epidemics. Other serious situations, which touch on problems of ethics, politics or social affairs, such as the cases of Zaire, Rwanda, Tibet or the Amazon Indians, have not been included this time.

Most of the populations covered in this book are facing life-threatening danger. The people of Sudan are arguably the most at risk as the country has one of the worst records of killings, organized starvation and deportations of civilians in recent history. In addition to a brutal war between the Sudanese army and the SPLA rebels in the south, internecine fighting within the SPLA has resulted in thousands of victims and tens of thousands of displaced people and refugees. Despite recent international pressure, relief efforts have long been hampered by the international community's diplomatic respect for a government with one of the worst human rights records on the African continent.

In the Caucasus, the fighting over Nagorno-Karabakh has now shifted into a new phase, resulting in more victims in twelve months than over the last four years. The conflict between Abkhazians and Georgians has flared up once again, as has the violence between the Ossetians and the Ingush. The international community's unwillingness to get bogged down in new territorial disputes means that Moscow has been given the green light for single-handed policing.

The Bosnian war has caused 200,000 deaths and left 2,300,000 refugees. It is ironic that in the light of this situation, the Security Council comes up with countless resolutions requesting the protection of populations and the setting up of security zones, while war criminals are welcomed in Geneva as respectable heads of state. Preoccupied by the current economic and monetary crisis, Europe has taken to using humanitarian aid as a cosmetic device which is allowing it to sit out the crisis until the ultimate cleansing produces a new manageable Bosnia, officially carved up along ethnic lines.

In Somalia, the international community, which, for two years, had been conspicuous by its absence, suddenly opted for military intervention under the flag of the United States in December 1992. Although better-protected convoys of humanitarian aid now reach former no-go areas, military concerns have completely overshadowed any fledgling political settlements and, ironically, have hampered the humanitarian effort.

Over the last months, four situations have given rise to heightened concern. The war which had been devastating the provinces of Afghanistan for fifteen years finally engulfed Kabul. Fighting between the various groups of Mujahideen has turned the capital into a wasteland to the total indifference of the international community. Once the focal point of the Cold War, Afghanistan has been abandoned to its fate.

In Tajikistan, the war sparked off by the short-lived takeover of power by the anti-communist opposition and the subsequent Moscow-backed clampdown killed 50,000 people and displaced 500,000. Often misconstrued in the West as a test ground for the spread of fundamentalism, the conflict, in fact, foreshadows the implosion of such Stalinist creations as the Tajik republic.

The intervention of West African countries in Liberia has in fact worsened the partisanship of the conflict. By taking sides against Charles Taylor – even to the extent of attacking humanitarian aid convoys and obstructing much-needed rescue operations – the ECOMOG 'peacekeeping force', which operates under the distant control of the UN, has become directly responsible for starving out and killing innocent civilians.

The Angolan peace process has given rise to a war more frightening than any during the Cold War. Having limited its objectives to the organization of 'free and fair' elections, without ensuring demobilization, the UN must bear the responsibility for one of today's most savage open conflicts.

The situations of Cambodia and El Salvador are slightly different in that recently some progress has been made, but they represent test cases in crisis intervention that this book cannot overlook. In these two countries, the international community has played an active role in paving the way for a political solution – albeit with varying degrees of success.

In El Salvador, confidence is slowly building up, allowing a demobilization of the armed forces and thorough human rights investigations. In Cambodia, however, the peace process remains tenuous, despite the success of the elections organized in May 1993. The threat of the continuing presence of the Khmer Rouge and the absence of systematic disarmament is casting a shadow over the country's chances of a return to peace.

Jacques de Milliano
Chairman, MSF International (1993)

AUTHORS AND ACKNOWLEDGEMENTS

PART 1

René Backmann, *Le Nouvel Observateur* magazine, Paris.
Roy Gutman, *Newsday* newspaper, New York.
Alain Hertoghe, *La Croix-L'évènement* newspaper, Paris.
François Jean, Médecins Sans Frontières, Paris.
Christine Messiant, Centre National de la Recherche Scientifique (CNRS), Paris.
Olivier Roy, CNRS, Paris.
Sophie Shihab, *Le Monde* newspaper, Paris.
Stephen Smith, *Libération* newspaper, Paris.
Joëlle Tanguy, Médecins Sans Frontières, Mogadishu.
Alex de Waal, African Rights, London.

PART 2

Philippe Biberson, Rony Brauman, Eric Goemaere, Guy Hermet, Jean-Christophe Rufin, Françoise Bouchet-Saulnier, all of Médecins Sans Frontières.

The text in boxes was written by Eric Dachy, Alain Destexhe, Myriam Gaume, Anne Guibert, Pierre Haski, Pierre Humblet, Michel Kassa, Guillaume Le Gallais, Dominique Martin, Frédérique Marodon, Bernard Pécoul, Marc Van den Berghe and Maurits Van Pelt.

English edition by Anne-Marie Huby and Alison Marschner.

AUTHORS AND ACKNOWLEDGEMENTS

Research and information by Marc Biot, Peter Casaer, Thierry Durand, Abdel-rahman Ghandour, Anne Guibert, Johan Heffinck, Karim Laouabdia, Sarah Khan, Etienne Krug, René Lataste, Nicolas Louis, Jean Rigal, Wilna Van Aartsen and Patrick Vial.

We would like to thank all representatives and volunteers of Médecins Sans Frontières in the field who provided vital information and precious support – as well as Jean-François Alesandrini, Rony Brauman, Alain Destexhe and Bernard Pécoul for their advice and comments.

ACRONYMS

AFL	Armed Forces of Liberia
ARENA	Alianza Republicana Nacional (El Salvador)
ASEAN	Association of South-East Asian Nations
CIS	Commonwealth of Independent States
CSCE	Conference on Security and Cooperation in Europe
DHA	United Nations Department of Humanitarian Affairs
ECOMOG	Economic Community Ceasefire Monitoring Group (Liberia)
ECOWAS	Economic Community of West African States
EC	European Community
FMLN	Frente Farabundo Marti para la Liberacion Nacional (El Salvador)
FUNCINPEC	United National Front for an Independent, Neutral, Peaceful and Cooperative Cambodia
ICRC	International Committee of the Red Cross
INPFL	Independent National Patriotic Front of Liberia
KPNLF	Khmer People's National Liberation Front
NATO	North Atlantic Treaty Organization
NGO	Non-Governmental Organization
NPFL	National Patriotic Front of Liberia
ONUSAL	United Nations Observer Mission in El Salvador
SNC	Supreme National Council (Cambodia)
SPLA	Sudan People's Liberation Army
SRPA	United Nations Special Relief Programme for Angola
ULIMO	United Liberation Movement for Democracy in Liberia
UNAVEM	United Nations Angola Verification Mission
UNDP	United Nations Development Programme
UNHCR	United Nations High Commissioner for Refugees
UNICEF	United Nations Children Fund
UNITA	National Union for the Total Independence of Angola

UNITAF	United Nations Task Force (Somalia)
UNOSOM	United Nations Operation in Somalia
UNPROFOR	United Nations Protection Force in former Yugoslavia
UNTAC	United Nations Transitional Authority in Cambodia
UNTAG	United Nations Transitional Arrangement Group (Namibia)
USAID	United States Agency for International Development
WFP	World Food Programme
WHO	World Health Organization

INTRODUCTION

The end of the Cold War raised again the idea of an international community based on shared values, administered by international institutions and defended by democratic countries. In the face of the increasing number of crises, the international community is regularly called upon to encourage negotiations, to interpose itself between factions and to assist people at risk. Although for years the great powers were vilified for exacerbating and protracting conflicts throughout the world, today all hopes are pinned on their involvement in the search for a political solution.

The United Nations, powerless during the Cold War as a result of the superpower hostility which essentially restricted its role to development aid, has now been given a real ability to take initiatives and is looking to develop its capability for emergency interventions in crisis situations.

A NEW ROLE FOR THE UN

The UN's return to centre stage, symbolized by the award of the Nobel Peace Prize to the Blue Helmets in 1988, can be seen in the dramatic increase in its activity. In the four years from 1988 to 1992, it has carried out more operations – thirteen in all – than in the preceding forty years and the number of Blue Helmets has increased from 10,000 to 52,000. Since then, the UN peacekeeping activities have continued to grow. By June 1993, the number of Blue Helmets had increased to 75,000, mainly owing to the intervention in Somalia, and no month goes by without a new operation starting up – in Rwanda, Georgia, Tajikistan or South Africa.

This boom in UN activity is in striking contrast to its past inertia. East–West confrontation paralysed the Security Council for forty years and prevented the implementation of the collective security system

1

provided for by the San Francisco Charter. The UN could not do much about the conflicts springing up in the shadow of superpower rivalry. It was limited to a narrowly constrained activity that was to become known as 'peacekeeping'. This improvised mechanism, which was not foreseen under the Charter and which Secretary-General Dag Hammarskjöld described as 'chapter six and a half', bridged the gap between Chapter VI, dealing with the peaceful resolution of conflicts, and Chapter VII, covering enforcement measures ranging from economic sanctions to the use of force to maintain international peace and security.

The basic principles of peacekeeping – the consent of the parties and the non-use of force, except in the last resort and in self-defence – clearly reflected the constraints involved in playing the Cold War zero-sum game. This meant, in effect, the symbolic deployment of observers or neutral forces between the warring parties, providing they had agreed to suspend hostilities in the first place. Essentially, this did little more than preserve the *status quo* and win time until a political solution, however unlikely, could be found.

Today, the observers have become players. The permanent members of the Security Council, who used and abused their right of veto for four decades, have finally begun to collaborate in the spirit of collegiality laid out in the Charter and are ready to play the game of multilateral diplomacy. The number of interventions has increased, as has the diversity of UN missions. As a result, peacekeeping has become a misleading concept, now covering a whole range of activities from mine clearing to organizing elections, demobilizing and disarming combatants, repatriating and reintegrating refugees, training police forces, defending human rights and rebuilding ruined economies.

The operations in 1990–1 in Angola, El Salvador and Cambodia were among the first illustrations of this newly extended field of intervention – albeit improvised in a way that has characterized peacekeeping since its inception. It is obvious, however, that these recent interventions have broken away from the parameters of traditional peacekeeping based on the deployment of Blue Helmets with the consent of the belligerents following a ceasefire or peace agreement. UN operations no longer aim solely at maintaining the *status quo,* as can be seen in its 1992 interventions in Bosnia and Somalia. Concern for stability has not diminished – indeed, it is stronger than ever – but it goes with a more dynamic interpretation of the role of the UN, as it is entrusted not only with peacekeeping as such but also with the restoration of law and order and the protection of humanitarian aid operations. The UN's role has never been so important – nor has it ever been so controversial.

SOVEREIGNTY AND INTERVENTION

Against this new background, the foundations of the UN appear all the more anachronistic. One of the major problems is that the UN system is based on the notion of state sovereignty. Chapter II(7) of the UN Charter stresses that a country's internal affairs are its exclusive concern. Although civil wars and internal strife account for most present-day conflicts, the Charter only covers wars erupting across frontiers between conventional armies. As a result, the mechanisms for collective security are in principle applicable only in international conflicts.

Today however, this conventional notion of state sovereignty, which was reaffirmed at the end of the Second World War, strengthened during the decolonization period and frozen by East–West confrontation, has become outdated. The end of the Cold War has had the dual effect of questioning the Yalta world order, sustained by the ideological blocs, and the principle of national sovereignty enshrined in the treaty of Westphalia.

The idea of the nation-state was already put into question in the 1970s, before the fall of the Berlin Wall began to show its first effects. The Helsinki Agreements eroded the principle of sovereignty by turning human rights into an issue of international concern. Many people had long lost faith in it anyway, their authoritarian rulers having discredited it beyond redemption.

Since then, it has continually been challenged. As the economies of the world have become increasingly integrated, so too have many other spheres, such as the media, the environment, migrations and humanitarian aid. Even the most repressive states have lost the ability to control the circulation of people and ideas. By contrast, the UN's respect for sovereignty makes it look like a bastion of tradition.

The human rights movement at the end of the 1980s prompted further attacks on sovereignty. The idea that regimes can commit large-scale human rights violations with impunity had become un-acceptable, as was evidenced by UN Secretary-General Javier Perez de Cuellar at the end of his term of office, who claimed: 'We are clearly witnessing what is probably an irresistible shift in public attitudes toward the belief that the defence of the oppressed in the name of morality should prevail over frontiers and legal documents'.

Respect for sovereignty remains all-important but in some instances calls for the protection of victims seem to have been heeded. Seen from that angle, there are common interventionist overtones in Security Council Resolution 688 condemning Iraq's repression of its civilian population – and insisting that humanitarian organizations have immediate access to them – Resolution 770 on the protection of humanitarian convoys in Bosnia and, finally, Resolution 794 on the use of force to restore security for aid operations in Somalia.

Each of these three resolutions on Iraq, Bosnia and Somalia are landmarks in the recent history of international intervention. While self-defence used to provide the only justification for intervention in an internal conflict – the Tanzanian intervention in Uganda and the Vietnamese invasion of Cambodia were presented in 1979 as a reply to outside aggression – humanitarian concerns are now put forward as the driving rationale behind the 'new interventionism'. Resolution 688 on Iraq was a first in that it linked humanitarian concerns to international peace and security on the ground of the mass exodus of refugees into neighbouring countries.

In Resolutions 770 on Bosnia and 794 on Somalia, which opened the way to interventions authorizing the use of force, in conformity with Chapter VII of the Charter, it is the crisis itself that was described as a threat to peace and security. Although the UN troops in Croatia took on a conventional peacekeeping mission – in fact guaranteeing the *status quo* in areas captured by Serbs – those who were finally deployed in the open war of Bosnia, after much procrastination, were called on to use 'all necessary means' to protect humanitarian convoys.

Similarly, in Somalia, the UN went from sending, almost discreetly, 50 observers and 500 Blue Helmets with the warlords' consent, to the non-negotiated deployment of 2,500 extra troops. This was followed by the landing of 30,000 GIs authorized to 'employ all necessary means to establish a secure environment for humanitarian relief operations', and finally, to the high-handed takeover of the country by 28,000 Blue Helmets, ready – and willing – to use force. The operations carried out in 1992 demonstrate the emergence, still hesitant and cautious in Bosnia, but more obvious and aggressive in Somalia, of new kinds of military intervention under humanitarian cover that are further removed from the traditional principles of peacekeeping.

INTRODUCTION

AT PAINS TO HANDLE INTERNAL CRISES

Despite these recent developments, caution remains the rule. The Security Council is still reluctant to consider even large-scale human rights violations as threats to international peace and security. However, decades of Cold War constraints and strict observance of non-interference alone cannot explain the UN's long-standing inability to intervene. The international community has obvious difficulty in acting in internal crises, usually quite complex and not susceptible to resolution by outside intervention. The UN can certainly play a vital role as arbitrator and guarantor when the warring parties agree to negotiate peace but in the absence of such an agreement, outside intervention can become part of the problem as much as it can bring a long-term solution – as was the case in the Congo from 1960 to 1964 and the Lebanon from 1982 to 1984, where the international forces rapidly became parties to the conflicts.

Roughly speaking, the international community is confronted with three types of crises: wars of aggression (Kuwait), large-scale human rights violations and repression of minorities (Burma) and the total collapse of law and order (Somalia). In none of these cases are there any easy answers, but the UN is aware that it must be ready to commit itself to the long and painstaking search for long-term solutions.

More importantly, the international community is obviously at pains to catch up with an ever-changing, seemingly chaotic world, where institutions are crumbling, armed forces are splitting up into factions and conflicts are tearing entire countries apart. Deprived of their former Cold War backers, both government forces and guerrilla movements in today's war spots are increasingly left to fend for themselves and forced to fight over the scant resources available. Obliged to depend on their own strength, they have to find new, and often brutal, ways of procuring weapons and consolidating power.

The majority of wars today have become 'privatized' concerns, financed by looting, racketeering and trafficking. The striking feature common to most present-day crisis situations is self-perpetuation of violence. It is true that the end of the Cold War opened new opportunities for negotiated solutions, but it has also lessened the possibilities for powerful countries to exert real pressure on the warring parties. Moreover, as trustworthy representatives and leaders are harder to find on the scenes of today's conflicts, it is all the more difficult to impose respect for international law. Laws that cannot be enforced only pave the way for lawlessness.

THE QUESTION OF INTERVENTION

Whatever the difficulties in intervening, the UN is faced with an irrepressible demand for action. But many questions remain open as to how best to intervene. Without doubt, the one condition for success is early deployment. In this regard, the developments of the past years reveal large gaps in the international community's ability to curtail the spiral of violence at an early stage before it spins entire societies into chaos. In the absence of international involvement, the Liberian conflict developed over six months into a frenzy of violence and massacres before a regional force intervened. In Somalia, the international community took almost two years to react, after having left the country prey to violence and starvation. In former Yugoslavia, the European Community hesitated, leaving the field free for the aggressors to pursue a policy of terror and 'ethnic cleansing' at the heart of Europe. From the Caucasus to Tajikistan, from Zaire to Rwanda, the much-debated policies of prevention are in fact mainly reactive and, more often than not, too late.

Consequently, the most pressing question too often concerns that of the last resort solution – military intervention. Although stepping in without the agreement of the warring parties becomes more and more common, the UN will have to adapt to a new set of rules for which it is still ill-prepared. Its ill-defined mandates and blatant shortcomings in coordinating various national contingents have seriously damaged its credibility and weakened the deterrent effect of the armed forces placed under its banner.

The UN aid agencies, too, have to improve their operational efficiency. Despite vague attempts at reform, the UN continues to be governed by inertia, lack of accountability, sometimes even incompetence, which hinder its ability to respond, especially to emergencies. Moreover, improved coordination between the different UN bodies is long overdue. The machinery is grinding to a halt as the myriad UN agencies too often function like private fiefdoms when the UN has to juggle peacekeeping, emergency relief and long-term recovery programmes all at once. In fairness however, the UN's ability to intervene ultimately depends on the political and financial backing of the member states, particularly in the West. The Secretary-General is probably right in saying that what cripples the organization most is too high expectations.

In the post-Cold War world, it is the countries of the West, led by the United States, which find themselves, by default, guarantors of the world order, although they are reluctant to act as an international police force. In the Gulf War the UN launched its biggest operation since the intervention in Korea to re-establish Kuwait's international borders, yet the coalition forces did nothing to defend the Shi'ites or the Kurds when they were violently supressed by Baghdad. It took the mass exodus across the frontiers of neighbouring countries to provoke an international intervention, which turned out to be little more than an after-sales service forced on the participants in order to safeguard the image of a 'just war'. It responded to public emotion and removed the threat of a massive influx of refugees into Turkey.

This half-hearted commitment to the Iraqi Kurds in a defeated country under international surveillance illustrates the reluctance of the West to get involved in internal crises. Faced with many crisis situations throughout the world, democratic countries are torn between defending human rights, i.e., contemplating intervention, and their reluctance to run the risks involved. The Security Council reflects the way the balance has tilted when it churns out resolutions without giving itself the means to enforce them.

The developments of the past two years have shattered all illusions of a new system of international protection that was supposedly heralded in Iraqi Kurdistan. More calls for help can be heard from oppressed people and minority groups, but Western countries have neither the financial and military clout, nor, above all, the political will to impose a new world order based on respect for human rights. The international community's response will only be prompted by political interests, media visibility and the sustained pressure of public opinion.

In short, Part 1 of *Life, Death and Aid* examines the four levels of international involvement in crisis situations: the complete absence from the scene of forgotten tragedies, intervention by regional powers, peacemaking operations in former Cold War battlegrounds and, finally, 'humanitarian' military interventions.

NON-INTERVENTION

For over a year, the highly-publicized UN operations in Bosnia, Somalia and Cambodia have overshadowed the lack of commitment to many other countries torn apart by war. Admittedly, these countries are not totally forgotten as humanitarian organizations and UN agencies struggle to bring aid to people at risk, despite insecurity and political obstacles. More often than not, international intervention is restricted to timid diplomatic overtures in these countries and, eventually, to economic pressures, but this does not guarantee genuine access to victims or an end to human rights violations. In Sudan and Afghanistan, the international community failed miserably to ensure that regular aid reach the threatened populations because it lacked real political commitment. Sudan, however, remains the harshest illustration of what amounts to 'non-assistance to populations in danger'.

REGIONAL INTERVENTION

The UN has been faced with so many requests for help over the past few years that the Secretary-General has been trying to encourage a more significant role for regional organizations in conflict resolution, according to Chapter VIII of the Charter. However, the problem has been to find credible partners. Many regional organizations are limited by a lack of ability, resources or political cohesion from taking part in peacekeeping operations. An example of this was the powerlessness of the Organization of African Unity (OAU) to deal either with the Somalian tragedy or any of the other recurring crises on the continent. However, the Organization of American States (OAS) and the European Community (EC) have demonstrated a degree of cooperation with the UN, albeit with mediocre results, in Haiti and former Yugoslavia.

Regional interventions have an obvious advantage in that they bring together the countries directly concerned and most likely to intervene, but their interests may not be purely altruistic: they do not always wait for the UN's invitation before interfering with their neighbours' problems. Syria intervened in Lebanon in 1976 under the guise of an Arab interposition force and, by playing a role akin to a pyromaniac fireman, succeeded in strengthening its grip on the country until its role was legitimized by the Taif agreements. In 1971, India intervened and precipitated the secession of its Pakistani rival by taking advantage of the large-scale human rights violations in East Pakistan and the arrival of millions of refugees across its borders. India, again, benefited from its regional supremacy in 1987, when it intervened in Sri Lanka on the pretext of bringing humanitarian aid to the Tamils. As for Vietnam's intervention in Cambodia in 1979, it put an end to the Khmer Rouge campaign of extermination but in essence it ensured Hanoi's domination of the Indo-Chinese peninsula.

There are many such ambiguities in the regional interventions launched over the past years. In Tajikistan, Russia, which controls the only organized armed forces in the republic, can hardly qualify as a peace guarantor as Moscow played a determining role in the communists' return to power. Ironically, Russia was readily given its peacekeeper credentials by an international community unwilling to get bogged down in the forgotten conflict. The deployment of a mixed intervention force in Ossetia and Abkhazia can hardly hide the central policing role played by Russia in the Caucasus conflicts. Here, Moscow has taken on the dual role of referee and player in its efforts to maintain its influence in the region, while looking for international backing.

Finally, Nigeria, which is the main backer of the West African intervention force in Liberia, argues, with the UN's blessing, that peace can only be attained by the crushing of one of the parties. Famine relief operations are hampered in the process, but then aid is in turn accused of hindering 'peace efforts'.

RESTORING PEACE IN THE RUINS OF THE COLD WAR

The end of the Cold War has opened up the possibility of resolving conflicts born in the shadow of superpower rivalry at the end of the 1970s. But these conflicts have deep local roots, structured around war economies that tend to perpetuate themselves, roots that go deeper than political and ideological differences.

In Central America, Southern Africa and South-East Asia, the former superpowers are involved in peace negotiations with UN help, with the special role of supervising their application in the field. In Salvador, Angola, Cambodia and, more recently, Mozambique, the UN has intervened to guarantee ceasefires, oversee disarmament, repatriate refugees, organize elections, rebuild infrastructures, etc. The success of such large-scale operations requires reliable support from member states at a time when the UN is in serious financial difficulties. It also requires effective coordination between the individual, but necessarily interdependent, aspects of these complex operations.

However, the principal problem relates to the difficulty of turning a diplomatic agreement into a political process. In El Salvador, it was the willingness of the former warring parties to reach an agreement that allowed the UN to act as a catalyst of the peace process. In Angola and Cambodia, on the contrary, the UN behaved as if its sole objective was to organize elections as planned.

'HUMANITARIAN' INTERVENTION

Further up the scale of intervention, humanitarian considerations have been pushed into the foreground in order to justify armed intervention in the face of a repressive regime (Iraq), a country subjected to aggression (Bosnia) or a collapsing state (Somalia). At first glance, there is no reason not to welcome this new international willingness to intervene, but putting good intentions into effect is a tricky task. Intervention in internal conflicts, without the agreement of the opposing sides, means that the international force can either favour negotiations at the risk of being taken hostage by one side or another, or it can opt for force and risk becoming yet another party to the conflict. The operations launched in 1992 are evidence of the difficulty of such interventions, characterized as they are by impotence in Bosnia where humanitarian aid has done more to allow than to hinder 'ethnic cleansing', and by aggression in Somalia where it was soon sidelined by sheer military might.

In both cases, the problem has been exacerbated by the absence of a clear political objective. In Bosnia, the humanitarian effort initially served as an alibi for the West's stand-off in the face of aggression before becoming another, more perverse, argument against military action, which might endanger troops deployed in the field. In Somalia, the use of force without clear political objectives made humanitarian aid one of the first casualties of war. As a result, the Blue Helmets have cast aside all pretence of impartiality and independence, thereby discrediting the entire international relief effort. Worst of all, the UN troops have violated the very principles of the Geneva Conventions by attacking hospitals and aid organizations.

This peace enforcement mission, the first ever for the UN, throws a particularly harsh light on the contradictions between the restoration of peace, which supposes a clearly defined political strategy, and humanitarian aid, which demands strict impartiality and independence. We hope that the UN impasse in Bosnia and Somalia will force a much-needed political debate on the principles and workings of future international interventions.

François Jean

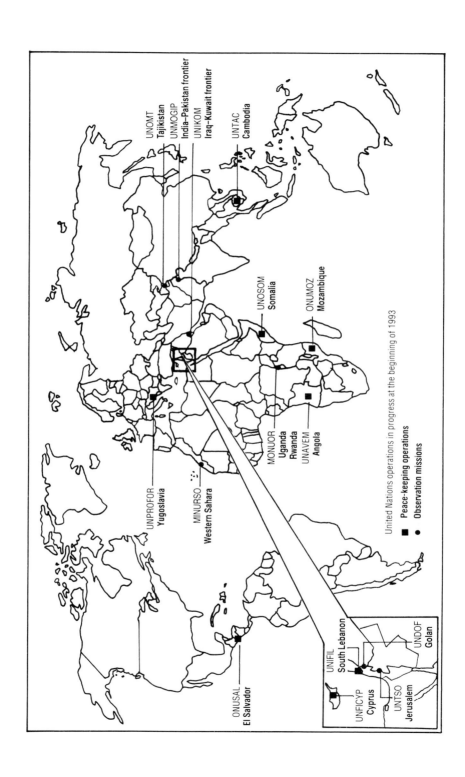

UNOMT
Tajikistan

UNMOGIP
India–Pakistan frontier

UNIKOM
Iraq–Kuwait frontier

UNTAC
Cambodia

UNOSOM
Somalia

ONUMOZ
Mozambique

MONUOR
Uganda
Rwanda

UNAVEM
Angola

UNPROFOR
Yugoslavia

MINURSO
Western Sahara

ONUSAL
El Salvador

UNIFIL
South Lebanon

UNFICYP
Cyprus

UNTSO
Jerusalem

UNDOF
Golan

United Nations operations in progress at the beginning of 1993

■   Peace-keeping operations
●   Observation missions

Peacekeeping operations (1945–88)

1956–7   UNEF 1, First United Nations Emergency Force
1958   UNOGIL, United Nations Observation Group in Lebanon
1960–4   ONUC, United Nations Operation in the Congo
1962–3   UNSF, United Nations Security Force in West New Guinea
1963–4   UNYOM, United Nations Yemen Observation Mission
1965–6   DOMREP, Mission of the Representative of the Secretary-General
         in the Dominican Republic
1965–6   UNIPOM, United Nations India–Pakistan Observation Mission
1973–9   UNEF 2, Second United Nations Emergency Force (Suez Canal,
         then Sinai)

Operations still underway

1948–   UNTSO, United Nations Truce Supervision Organization (Palestine)
1949–   UNMOGIP, United Nations Military Observer Group in
         India and Pakistan
1964–   UNFICYP, United Nations Peacekeeping Force in Cyprus
1974–   UNDOF, United Nations Disengagement Observer Force (Golan)
1978–   UNIFIL, United Nations Interim Force in Lebanon

Operations launched by the UN since 1988

1988–90 UNGOMAP, United Nations Good Offices Mission in Afghanistan
         and Pakistan
1988–91 UNIIMOG, United Nations Iran–Iraq Military Observer Group
1989–91 UNAVEM 1, United Nations Angola Verification Mission 1
1989–90 UNTAG, United Nations Transition Assistance Group (Namibia)
1989–92 ONUCA, United Nations Observer Group in Central America
1991–   UNIKOM, United Nations Iraq–Kuwait Observation Mission
1991–   ONUSAL, United Nations Observer Mission in El Salvador
1991–   MINURSO, United Nations Mission for the Referendum
         in Western Sahara
1991–2   UNAMIC, United Nations Advance Mission in Cambodia
1992–   UNPROFOR, United Nations Protection Force in former Yugoslavia
1992–   UNTAC, United Nations Transitional Authority in Cambodia
1992–   UNAVEM 2, United Nations Angola Verification Mission 2
1992–3   UNOSOM 1, United Nations Operation in Somalia 1

1992–   UNOMSA United Nations Observer Mission in South Africa
1992–   UNOMOZ, United Nations Operation in Mozambique
1993–   UNOSOM 2, United Nations Operation in Somalia 2
1993–   MONUOR, United Nations Observer Mission in Uganda
         and Rwanda
1993–   UNOMT, United Nations Observer Mission in Tajikistan

Part 1

FROM ABSTENTION TO INTERVENTION – THE TEN CASES

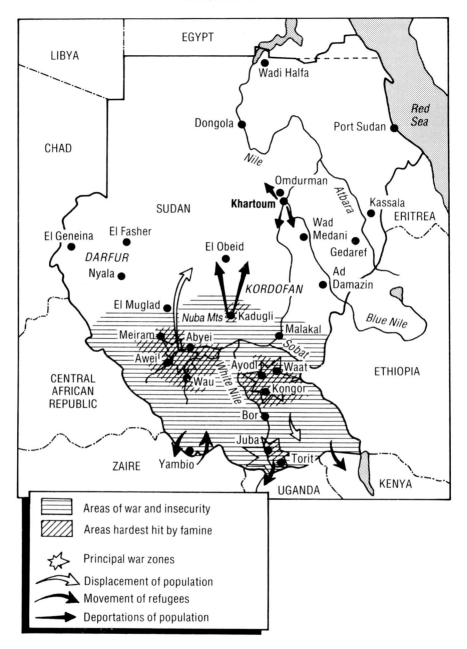

Areas of war and insecurity

Areas hardest hit by famine

Principal war zones

Displacement of population

Movement of refugees

Deportations of population

1

SUDAN
Speak no evil, do no good

The people of Sudan are suffering one of the gravest and most enduring human crises in the world. Since the outbreak of the civil war in 1983, writers have run out of adjectives to describe the calamities that have engulfed the country. Once hailed as the 'breadbasket of the Arab world', Sudan has been stricken by a succession of famines, which have profoundly disrupted the country's rural communities. Real incomes have plummeted. Formerly one of the most liberal and democratic countries in Africa and the Middle East, it is now ruled by a ruthless dictatorship that violates every human right in the book. Civil institutions have been destroyed, and the social services and health infrastructures have disintegrated, contributing to devastating epidemics of malaria, meningitis and kala-azar.

THE UN PARALYSIS

The war, fought mostly in the south, has been extraordinarily brutal and divisive, with tens of thousands of people killed by the army, government-armed militias and the factions of the rebel Sudan People's Liberation Army (SPLA). All sides are to blame. In the last two years, internecine fighting within the SPLA has been the largest cause of civilian deaths.

The war-famines have wreaked a death toll in the hundreds of thousands. They have also driven millions of people from their homes; most are congregated around the northern cities. This massive social crisis has been deepened by a government programme of forced relocation that is as large and brutal as any implemented in South Africa or Iraqi Kurdistan.

One of the most bitter tragedies of Sudan is that the dilemmas facing humanitarian organizations today are almost exactly those faced repeatedly over the last ten years. A decade's worth of experience includes a few successes and many failures. But while the generals and guerrillas have learned their lessons, the UN humanitarian agencies have not.

The Sudan government is heavily indebted and internationally ostracized. Despite this weak position, it has skilfully manipulated donor countries to keep control over humanitarian programmes. Throughout the 1980s, the United States, European Community and United Nations vied with each other for influence in Sudan. Each donor wanted the largest programmes, and each made major compromises to obtain them.

NO SUPPORT AT THE TOP

These compromises scuttled the best hopes for famine relief. In 1986, a group of NGOs pressed donor governments for improved aid to the south. They argued that aid should go to civilians on both sides, and should be accounted for, to reduce rates of diversion. The then-head of UNDP in Khartoum, Winston Prattley, endorsed this line, and formulated Operation Rainbow. The government vetoed the plan, accused Prattley of 'meddling in politics' and ordered him out of the country. The expulsion of the most senior UN official in the country was an unprecedented step – but neither the UN Secretariat, the USA nor the EC made more than a token protest. In fact, the EC was consigning food relief directly to the Sudanese army. The expulsion of Prattley sent an unmistakable signal: there was no support at the top for UN staff who tried to bend the rules to feed the hungry.

For the next two years, almost no food relief moved. Sudan received huge donations of food aid, but the government ensured that very little of it actually reached the hungry in the south, suspected of supporting the SPLA. An exceptionally severe famine developed: at its nadir in mid-1988, in the displaced camps of southern Kordofan, famine victims were dying at the rate of 1 per cent per day. Had it not been for a constant influx of more refugees, camps such as el Meiram, Abyei and Muglad would simply have become graveyards. Meanwhile, EC-donated food stood in railway wagons for more than two years, just a few hundred metres away.

The major donors sent nothing to SPLA-held areas. UNICEF started a modest programme to assist NGOs operating cross-border from Kenya but when the government objected, the UN obligingly closed it down.

In early 1989, the impasse was dramatically broken when a breakthrough in peace negotiations between Sadiq el Mahdi's government

Operation Lifeline Sudan

Operation Lifeline was a pioneering relief programme which is often presented as a model for humanitarian relief to war-stricken areas. The plan provided for relief to cross from government-held into rebel-held areas, and vice versa, in 'corridors of tranquillity' where military action was prohibited.

Although the UN was formally in charge of the operation, it was in fact the work of a broad range of agencies, mostly NGOs, working together under informal rules of cooperation. In its first phase, Operation Lifeline aimed to deliver 100,000 tonnes of food relief to southern Sudan in six months. It succeeded. This was a small part of the total needs but by the end of the year, the famine was conquered.

Because it is so often held up as a model, phase one of Operation Lifeline deserves scrutiny. Exactly why did it succeed? Two facts stand out as crucially important.

One is that the deal was struck as part of ongoing peace talks between the government and the SPLA. At the time, the peace process was forging ahead in such a way that neither side was looking to manipulate the programme to its military advantage.

The second is that the peace process rapidly brought about a general ceasefire. For the first time since the war began, this allowed people to return to their fields to plant, to cultivate in the confidence of reaping their crops, to herd their cattle freely, and to restart trade. The revival of the rural economy during the ceasefire made a huge contribution to people's survival – a contribution much greater than that made by the relief food itself.

By contrast, the later phases of Operation Lifeline during 1990–3, in the context of renewed fighting, failed to prevent a return of famine conditions, despite the sustained delivery of large amounts of food. The lesson of Operation Lifeline is that material relief alone cannot solve the humanitarian problems of a war-affected region. Food relief cannot substitute for a ceasefire which allows people to assist themselves.

and the SPLA and the new US policy of firmness towards Sudan allowed the UN to extricate itself from years of compliance with the Sudanese government. The result was Operation Lifeline Sudan, launched in April 1989, with the promise of taking relief to civilians on both sides of the battle lines in the south. It was a ground-breaking initiative in which a sovereign government formally agreed to a cross-border operation into rebel-held territory. This was the same formula as Operation Rainbow – three years and perhaps 250,000 lives later.

Sadly, Operation Lifeline failed to live up to its early promise. Along with the hopes of peace, it crumbled. In June 1989, the Sadiq government was overthrown in a military coup led by General Omer al Bashir. The new fundamentalist government launched new military offensives in the south and embarked upon the systematic trans-formation of the north into an Islamic state.

FOOD AS A WEAPON OF WAR

Operation Lifeline has continued. But gradually it has become an instrument of war, rather than a force for peace. The government has sought to wrest control of the operation, for instance by demanding that it has the right to approve all flight plans, including those to SPLA-held areas. It has been able to do this because instead of dealing with an array of NGOs, it has had to deal with only a single, compliant partner: the UN.

In the early days of Operation Lifeline, the UN was merely *primus inter pares* among the relief agencies, but it has gradually taken on a more formal coordinating role. For three years, the UN has held monthly negotiations with the government concerning which places can be reached, and prevaricates until the last moment before ap-proving the flight plans. Each time, the government pushes for its favoured destinations – its own garrison towns – to be the first beneficiaries. How much of the food goes to the army, no one knows.

The Sudan government has perfected the diplomatic art of beguiling the UN. It charms senior officials. It plays the donors off against each other. It offers just enough to tempt the UN – then delivers much less. It threatens to stop the whole programme if it is not appeased.

The SPLA also plays a sinister game with relief food. For many years it has fed its troops from international aid. UN food simply disappeared into vast refugee camps in western Ethiopia, with no accountability. In the south itself, some NGOs argued that if the SPLA soldiers were not fed, they would just plunder the local population.

Sudanese epidemic defies UN health agency

The kala-azar epidemic, which has wiped out entire communities displaced by the war in southern Sudan, has, over the past two years, illustrated the inability of the World Health Organization (WHO) to put humanitarian concerns before good relations with governments.

In December 1991, Sudanese researchers in Bentiu, a southern garrison town, carried out an evaluation of kala-azar. Their conclusions were alarming: an epidemic was seen to be threatening more than 18,000 people in greater Bentiu. The proposal to install a treatment centre was initially well received by the local WHO representative. However, he suddenly began to backpedal when confronted by opposition from the Sudanese government, which, despite the incredulous protests of local authorities, denied the existence of any epidemic whatsoever in the south of the country.

At the WHO headquarters in Geneva, kala-azar specialists were aware of the epidemic, but the alarming reports which reached them from the western province of the Upper Nile continued to go unheeded as long as the Khartoum office chose to do nothing. It was not until 1993, when the Nairobi office of UNICEF issued an alarming press release on the epidemic, that the United Nations finally began to talk about kala-azar in terms of a serious threat to public health in southern Sudan. Nevertheless, the local UNICEF office in Khartoum was quick to contradict the declarations of their colleagues in Kenya.

The WHO has proved to be doubly inefficient. On the one hand, while the local office enjoys great autonomy, the WHO headquarters cannot intervene locally even in a major crisis. On the other hand, the kala-azar crisis in southern Sudan illustrates the tendency of the United Nations to avoid opposing governments, even when this policy runs counter to the vital needs of the population. At a time when blind respect for the principle of sovereignty is tending to fade in the face of demands for aid and the defence of human rights, it is time for this sort of custom to change.

But often the SPLA still plundered the locals anyway. After the SPLA split in August 1991, the contending factions have used relief supplies to attract civilians to the areas they control, and to keep them there, while denying relief to the other side. The precedence of military over humanitarian values in the SPLA was graphically shown in September 1992, when SPLA soldiers murdered three expatriate aid workers in a still unexplained incident.

An incident in July 1992 illustrated not only how food relief became a weapon of war, but how an ineffectual UN response could endanger the whole humanitarian programme. The army hired Iliushin planes, previously used by the WFP to fly relief to Juba, for arms deliveries. The planes still had the WFP insignia on them – opening the UN up to the SPLA accusation that it was allowing its planes to be used to ferry weapons. The SPLA had often shot down planes with less justification. The UN sent a private *démarche*, which the Sudan government ignored. Arms flights continued for ten days, until WFP employees were able to scrape the insignia off the planes themselves. Still the UN said nothing in public. Presumably the UN felt that its relief programmes would be endangered by offending the government.

Around the same time, two UN employees were executed by the security forces in Juba, as part of a massacre following an SPLA attempt to storm the town. Again, the UN issued no public condemnation.

INTERNATIONAL PRESSURE AT LAST

By contrast, a resolute – even heavy-handed – US approach brought results. After two USAID employees were killed in Juba, in similar circumstances to the UN staff, the US government protested strongly. Congress passed a resolution condemning Sudan shortly afterwards. After the US military intervened in Somalia, there were implicit threats of similar action in southern Sudan.

Then, unexpectedly, the UN also took a firm line. This did not come from the Department of Humanitarian Affairs or the Secretariat, but from the unlikeliest sources – the General Assembly and the Human Rights Commission. On 2 December 1992, the General Assembly overwhelmingly voted to censure Sudan's human rights record, and a special *rapporteur* on human rights was appointed. The *rapporteur*, Gustav Biro, took his task seriously and compiled a damning report.

Under the growing pressure, the Sudan government became amenable. An opportunity similar to early 1989 opened up. The government agreed to UN proposals to deliver food to a long list of sites in the south, and began to negotiate on a proposal to create a demilitarized zone in the areas worst hit by the famine. It seemed as though Operation Lifeline was to be rejuvenated.

For two reasons, the opportunity was squandered. One was the continuing bitter infighting in the SPLA: the different factions could not agree on any proposals for demilitarized zones or unhindered delivery of relief. The other was the donors' preoccupation with sending food, in the absence of a broader strategy for achieving peace.

MASS DEPORTATIONS: THE UN REMAINS SILENT

The picture is further complicated by the fact that the war is not confined to the south. Since the beginning of the conflict, millions of southerners have fled to the north, many of them to the outskirts of Khartoum. Here they have been living in appalling conditions, some of them literally on rubbish tips. Fearing that the displaced could form a 'fifth column' in the capital for the SPLA, in 1991 the government began a programme of forced relocation – which also affected rural northerners displaced by drought. By the middle of 1992, the homes of perhaps 700,000 people had been bulldozed and burned. The people were relocated to ironically named 'Peace villages' at a distance from the city, where no housing or services were provided. During most of the programme, international agencies were denied access.

Throughout this massive violation, the UN was silent, confined by a self-imposed impotence. Though the UN never expressed support for the demolitions, it never condemned them. At the outset, it agreed to join a government-convened relocations committee. Against the advice of its own experts, time and again, the UN negotiated with the government for minor modifications to the programme – small improvements in humanitarian access or brief suspensions of the demolitions. The government made many promises, and broke them all. The UN even put forward a proposal to fund a model relocation project. Meanwhile the removals proceed unchecked. By the time the UN realized it had been duped, the demolitions were a *fait accompli*.

The war also spread to the Nuba Mountains of northern Sudan in the late 1980s. The Nuba are a minority non-Arab people in the north, traditionally the victims of discrimination. About a million strong, they speak a variety of vernacular languages and many of them practise traditional religions or Christianity. In 1987, the SPLA sent a battalion

23

to the Nuba Mountains, which had little difficulty in recruiting dis-affected young men. In response, the government armed local Arab militias.

Since then the area has been convulsed in a spiral of violence. The militia burned dozens of villages and killed thousands of civilians, but did not achieve their expected victory. In 1991, educated Nuba and community leaders began to 'disappear' at the hands of the security forces. In 1992, the army declared a *jihad* and began the most exten-sive and brutal actions to date, culminating in the forced removal of tens of thousands of Nuba from their homeland to camps further north, where about 100,000 people have been regrouped under heavy army surveillance. Hunger and disease are rampant. Their land has since been turned over to mechanized farms. The campaign has aptly been described as 'ethnic cleansing'.

The Nuba Mountains presented the UN's greatest challenge: a remote, closed area that is not in the south and thus does not fall under Operation Lifeline. A tough, creative approach was required. Excepting the harsh words from Gustav Biro in 1993, the UN has done little and said nothing. Jan Eliasson, head of the Department of Humanitarian Affairs, visited Sudan in September 1992 but declined to make any public comment on the abuses: he said that human rights fell outside his mandate.

Challenged on these questions, UN staff have alibis: they did their jobs according to the rules. The rules lay out respect for national sovereignty and working only with the permission of the host govern-ment. And those who put humanitarian principles first, thus breaking with the sacrosanct principle of sovereignty, like Prattley, paid with their jobs. In the face of massive human rights violations and official determination to hamper relief efforts for the most threatened popu-lations, the UN simply stuck to its ordinary operating procedures in an extraordinary situation. It was consistently pusillanimous, and as a result became party to a huge and needless tragedy.

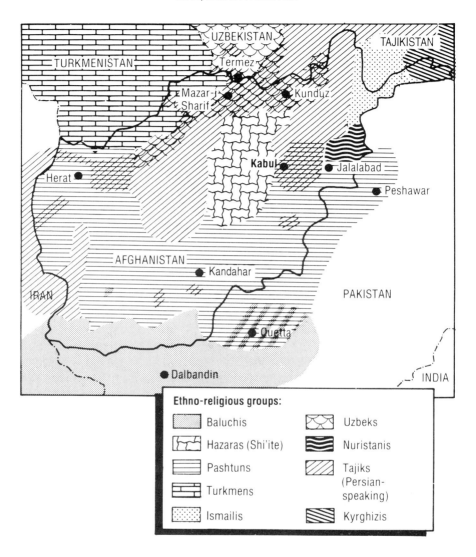

Ethno-religious groups:

Baluchis		Uzbeks	
Hazaras (Shi'ite)		Nuristanis	
Pashtuns		Tajiks (Persian-speaking)	
Turkmens			
Ismailis		Kyrghizis	

2

AFGHANISTAN
Off the agenda

Afghanistan has been devastated by war for over fifteen years. It is a conflict that marked a turning point in the Cold War: the Soviet invasion in December 1979 signalled the end of *détente* and the height of the Soviet threat, whereas the withdrawal of the expeditionary force in January 1989 meant the end of East–West confrontation and the collapse of the Soviet empire. The departure of the Red Army, however, was not enough to restore peace to the country and the fighting that has continued since 1989 has claimed heavy casualties although Afghanistan no longer makes the headlines. The country provides a sad example of a conflict born out of the Cold War, dragging on interminably and taking on a life of its own amidst widespread indifference.

FROM *JIHAD* TO ETHNIC FIGHTING

War in Afghanistan broke out in 1978 when the communist People's Democratic Party of Afghanistan, which had staged a coup and seized power on 27 April, launched a number of radical reforms coupled with a violent crackdown on traditional power groups. This policy turned most of the largely rural population, traditionally distrustful of central power and deeply attached to Islam, into armed opponents: within a few months the rebels controlled two-thirds of the country. The repression was ferocious but ineffective and the regime was about to collapse when the Soviet Union decided to intervene.

The invasion of Afghanistan on 27 December 1979 by over 100,000 combat troops supported by considerable air power precipitated the whole country into all-out war. The military outcome was uncertain, as the army was facing an elusive enemy and a deeply hostile population, but purges led to massive population displacements and the flight of millions of refugees into Pakistan and Iran. In a few months

Pakistan became host to the largest refugee population in the world. From 1984 intensified fighting speeded up the exodus: hundreds of villages were bombed, irrigation systems destroyed, the Panjshir valley emptied of almost all its inhabitants, the suburbs of Herat razed to the ground. And yet, despite all their efforts, the Soviet troops did not succeed in cutting off the supply lines to the resistance fighters and breaking the opposition. In February 1988 Mikhail Gorbachev announced the withdrawal of the expeditionary force and the last Soviet troops left Afghanistan in February 1989. To everyone's surprise, Najibullah's regime did not fall immediately: his policy, based on clever manipulation of ethnic and tribal divisions, met with relative success and enabled him to stay in power until the break-up of the Soviet Union in the autumn of 1991. In spring 1992, General Dostam, leader of the pro-communist Uzbek troops, did an about–turn and allied himself with Massud, one of the cleverest resistance commanders, and Kabul fell into the hands of the Mujahideen. Since the fall of Najibullah the fighting has moved towards the capital and pits the 'northerners' (Tajiks and Uzbeks) against the troops of Gulbuddin Hikmatyar, essentially Pashtuns, with the Shia Hazaras fighting their own corner. The *jihad* against Soviet power and the communists has given way to a civil war opposing the various ethnic and religious segments of Afghan society.

A SOCIETY ADRIFT

In fifteen years of war more than a million people have lost their lives and social structures have been shattered. Over a third of the Afghan population, estimated at fifteen million before the war, has sought refuge abroad, mostly in Pakistan but also in Iran, and hundreds of thousands have had to leave their villages and seek shelter in the outskirts of the towns. It is now the turn of the people of Kabul, largely spared while under Soviet occupation, to seek refuge outside the capital, which has become the battlefield for Mujahideen groups fighting over the remains of a state long since dead.

This extraordinary upheaval has had far-reaching effects on the country's social structure. A whole generation of young Afghans was born in refugee camps abroad or brought up in the mountains, in Mujahideen bases, and no longer knows how to farm. Traditional figures of authority (mullahs, landowners, tribal aristocracy), already decimated under the communist regime, have been replaced by young military commanders, sometimes well educated, who owe their power to their weapons or their ability to plug into an international

28

circuit of 'goods', be they weapons, trade, drugs or humanitarian aid. Traditional ways to settle conflicts, calling upon the elders or 'white beards', have lost their appeal, especially since the excessive number of arms in the country turns the slightest disagreement into carnage. The state machinery has disintegrated and schools and the few health facilities have been destroyed.

Whereas the rural population has been deeply affected by the war against the Soviets, it is now the turn of city-dwellers to become the victims of civil war between the Mujahideen: the capital, divided into 'ethnic areas', is torn apart by the endless settling of old scores against a background of violent crime. The efforts of the Hizbe-Islami to evict Massud from Kabul claimed many victims by heavy fire from multiple rocket launchers. Over a two-week period in August, a rain of rockets fell on the city, killing 1,000 people and forcing 300,000 to flee. Following a fragile ceasefire signed in September, fighting resumed with unprecedented intensity in January. There were 2,000 people killed and more than 10,000 wounded, only a minority of whom could be treated in the few hospitals spared by the attacks. Between bombings, the inhabitants strove to survive in a city strangled by a blockade which, in the winter of 1992–3, led to severe shortages of food and fuel. People fled the city in their thousands or wandered from one sector to another to escape fighting and shelling. Gulbuddin Hekmatyar's appointment as Prime Minister has not stopped the fighting, which is slowly turning the capital into a heap of rubble open to looting, random fire and epidemics caused by the lack of drinking water and the destruction of health facilities.

THE CONSTRAINTS OF THE COLD WAR

From its early beginnings to the withdrawal of the Soviet army, war in Afghanistan should be seen in the context of the Cold War and the so-called 'peripheral' disputes, in which the superpowers confronted one another through their regional proxies. The involvement of the Red Army ruled out open intervention on the part of the United States, which might have resulted in direct confrontation with disastrous consequences. Thus, US involvement was limited to clandestine support for the Mujahideen channelled through the Pakistani military and secret services.

With one of the permanent members of the UN Security Council directly involved in the combat, the organization's efforts were severely hampered by the superpower rivalry. Its only, meagre, achievement was the organization in Geneva under the aegis of the Secretary-

General of indirect negotiations between Kabul and Islamabad, from which the Mujahideen were excluded. It was not until the USSR's change of heart and the signing in Geneva in April 1988 of an agreement on the withdrawal of Soviet troops that the negotiations produced any results.

The UN's humanitarian activities were likewise limited by the need to deal with a government hostile to any assistance in 'rebel areas', regardless of the fact that they were completely deprived and devastated by war. Most UN aid was therefore directed at the refugee camps, where the UNHCR, backed by the West, was very active.

The International Committee of the Red Cross (ICRC), which was also unable to become involved in areas controlled by the Mujahideen without the government's agreement, found itself able to act only in Kabul and Pakistan, where it set up hospitals to treat war victims and continued – without much success – its efforts to have prisoners of war released.

From 1979 to 1989, it was non-governmental organizations that ran most relief activities for the Afghan population, often brushing aside diplomatic considerations to do so. Most of the relief organizations concentrated on the refugee camps, but a few operated secretly inside the country, helping those sections of the population under greatest threat. The contribution of such organizations, over and above their material assistance, was in achieving media coverage by drawing attention to the plight of the people trapped by the fighting and by helping journalists gain access to the interior of the country. From 1984 onwards, new, Muslim, organizations began to be set up, more often than not with the financial backing of Saudi Arabia. They deliberately sought to counter the cultural influence of their western counterparts.

DESERTION BY THE INTERNATIONAL COMMUNITY

The pullout of Soviet troops, completed by 15 February 1989, radically changed the situation. The countries of the West, motivated essentially by their battle against the Soviet Union, gradually withdrew, leaving the United Nations to cope with the political and humanitarian aftermath. Afghanistan receded gradually into memory. In February 1989 hundreds of journalists gathered in Kabul to witness the predicted collapse of the Najibullah regime. A few of them returned in 1992 when it actual took place. The media has since grown tired of a conflict that had no apparent objective and the public lost interest in the Afghan question. Russia disavowed a continuity with the Soviet Union, and refused to countenance any responsibility for the destruction caused by the war. The United States simply withdrew, after an abortive attempt to recover the most sophisticated of its weapons, such as the Stinger missiles. The United Nations, left in the lurch by the great powers, proved unable to set up a coalition government in the period between the Soviet withdrawal and the taking of Kabul by the Mujahideen. Still pinning its hopes on a negotiated settlement, the UN was still attempting to set up a coalition government that would have included many members of the communist regime. The UN was taken by surprise when Kabul fell into the hands of the Mujahideen from the interior, whom they had systematically ignored in favour of the regime and the Peshawar parties. This failure is explained mainly by the UN's tendency to deal only with representatives of the government, at the risk of negotiating with non-representative people and losing touch with reality. Throughout the Afghan crisis, the UN overestimated its political influence. With regard to humanitarian aid, however, the UN innovated by creating the flexible Operation Salam, to help rebuild the country by working, in collaboration with NGOs, in stable regions, without waiting for a global political solution. However, until it was wound up in December, the initiative suffered from a lack of trust on the part of the Mujaideen leaders who accused the UN of supporting the regime in Kabul and who did not understand the split between the humanitarian and the political efforts. In August 1992, the violence in Kabul caused the last remaining Western embassies to close and the UN representatives to pack up and leave. Kabul today is in the situation that Mogadishu was in at the beginning of 1991: only a handful of relief organizations remain to tell the tale of the capital's tragedy and to attempt to help those trapped by the fighting.

This means that the only foreign presence to be found in Afghanistan is that of the regional powers: Pakistan, Iran and Uzbekistan, with Saudi Arabia in the background. Pakistan, Iran and Uzbekistan, which have borders with Afghanistan, are not keen to see a strong nationalist government emerge to threaten their regional ambitions. A sort of consensus has been forged, with each of Afghanistan's neighbours retaining a presence there by using an ethnic or religious group as a proxy – the Shia Hazaras for Tehran, the Uzbeks for Tashkent and some of the Pashtuns for Islamabad. In the light of Pakistan's leading role on the political scene in Kabul, Iran and Uzbekistan confine themselves to retaining indirect control over the border areas and backing their protégés in Kabul. This game among the regional powers is complicated by the active presence of Muslim, Arab and

Pakistani militants, who are working to promote the Muslim radicals in Kabul and who hold sway over the refugees in Kunduz, who have fled the neo-communist backlash in Tajikistan. This Muslim influence is channelled both through armed gangs made up of Arab volunteers and through Muslim NGOs wielding a direct political influence.

The UNHCR, the ICRC and a few Western humanitarian organizations are continuing their efforts, but are coming up against the open hostility of foreign Muslim groups and the widespread insecurity in many parts of the country. Following the murder of four UNHCR staff in February 1993 near Jalalabad, the UN decided to withdraw temporarily its personnel from the east and south of the country. However, Afghanistan does have some relatively stable regional powers, such as that maintained in Herat by Ismail Khan, where Western relief efforts are able to continue. Other than security problems, the UN activities are constrained by the lack of financial support from western countries. This has been particularly problematic as regards the repatriation of refugees. One year after the fall of Kabul, about one million refugees returned from Pakistan and several hundred thousand from Iran; the UNHCR lacks the means to facilitate their reintegration to their homelands, most of which are devastated by the war and covered in mines.

It would be an exaggeration to describe Afghanistan as returning to some kind of tradition of anarchy and civil war. The country was stable, if weak, from 1880 to 1978, with a break from 1928 to 1930. Today's chaos stems from a combination of ten years of war, ethnic strife, a surfeit of weapons, the inability of Mujahideen fighters to return to civilian life, drugs and arms trafficking and, above all, the direct intervention of the regional powers. Peace in Afghanistan depends less on an increased international involvement than on the complete withdrawal of the regional powers.

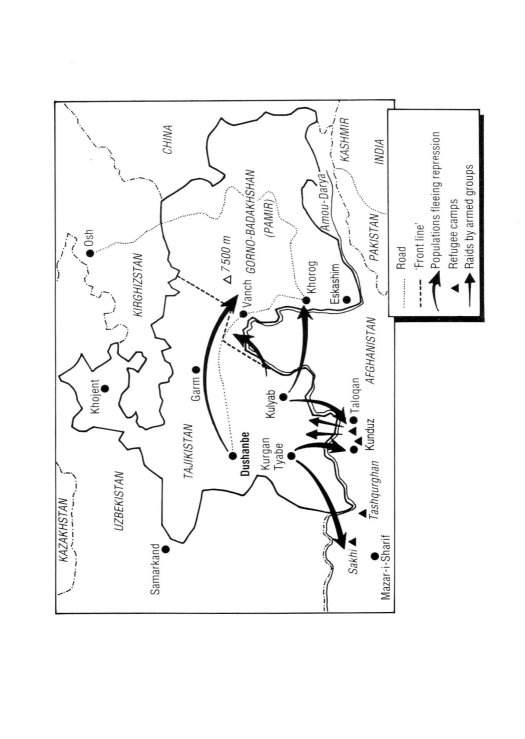

KAZAKHSTAN

UZBEKISTAN

KIRGHIZSTAN

Osh

Khojent

TAJIKISTAN

Garm

Samarkand

Dushanbe

Kulyab

Kurgan Tyabe

CHINA

△ 7 500 m

Vanch GORNO-BADAKHSHAN (PAMIR)

Khorog

Eskashim

Amou-Darya

KASHMIR

INDIA

PAKISTAN

AFGHANISTAN

Taloqan

Kunduz

Tashqurghan

Sakhi

Mazar-i-Sharif

Road

'Front line'

Populations fleeing repression

Refugee camps

Raids by armed groups

3

TAJIKISTAN
Free rein to the regional referees

Tajikistan became independent in October 1991 and was thrown virtually straight away into a state of internal turmoil. The toppling of the ruling Communist Party by a Muslim/democrat coalition in May 1992 gave way to a violent civil war which claimed tens of thousands of victims and put to flight hundreds of thousands of refugees and displaced persons. The return to power in December 1992 of pro-ponents of the old regime brought bloody repression, which was greeted with complete indifference by the international community. Since then, there has been no let-up in the fighting between the opposition – refugees in Afghanistan and the Pamir mountains – and the government, backed both by Uzbekistan, Tajikistan's powerful neighbour, and Russia, which controls the only regular troops in the Republic and now faces renewed problems with Afghanistan.

AN IDENTIKIT REPUBLIC

Tajikistan is the poorest of the republics resulting from the break-up of the USSR. Officially, it is 60 per cent Tajik, 20 per cent Uzbek and 20 per cent Russian; most of the Russians have left since the 1989 census was conducted, particularly since the unrest began and pro-voked a mass exodus of Europeans. The official census records several hundred thousand Ismailis among the Tajiks. Although the Ismailis are counted as Tajiks, they speak their own languages, and make up the majority of the population of the autonomous region of Gorno-Badakhshan in the Pamir mountains.

Like many of the former Soviet Republics, Tajikistan is a Stalinist invention. This explains many of its present problems. The Tajiks do not really exist as an ethnic group: they are the Persian-speaking Sunnis of Central Asia set apart from their neighbours by language. They have never been concentrated in a single area: Persian was the language of those who lived in the towns and foothills, while the plains and oases were 'Uzbekized' over the centuries. They never had a state of their own, even though Persian was the official language of most of the Uzbek emirates which dominated the region from the fifteenth to the nineteenth centuries. Establishing the Republic of Tajikistan thus amounted to inventing a territorial unit and building an ethnic or national identity around a language, Tajik, which resembles the Persian spoken in Iran and parts of Afghanistan. It was made the national language and given a Cyrillic alphabet. Tajikistan began life as an autonomous republic within Uzbekistan in 1925, and did not become a fully-fledged Soviet Republic until 1929. Samarkand and Bukhara, the cities which were the hubs of 'Tajik' civilization, ended up outside Tajikistan's borders, in Uzbekistan.

Cut off from their Persian roots and cultural elite, the people of Soviet Tajikistan began to identify more and more closely with the valleys and districts in which they lived. The key to this political game was a kind of parochialism, an allegiance to one's own area, a loyalty which transcended ideology, as was demonstrated by the Communist Party apparatchiks' tendency to promote those from their own village or region. The people who profited most from this in Soviet times were the natives of Khojent (ex-Leninabad), in the north of Tajikistan. All the First Secretaries of the Tajik Communist Party were from the area. In the 1970s, the Khojentis formed an alliance with the Kulyabis, the natives of the district of Kulyab, on the Afghan border. When it invaded Afghanistan, the USSR promoted Ismailis into the security forces, fearing that the Tajiks might feel sympathy for their Afghan brothers. This was not well received by the Khojentis or the Kulyabis. It was the other areas, which were deprived of power, that came to form the basis of the Islamic opposition.

While the communist cadres were unshakeable in their loyalty to Moscow, Tajikistan was one of the parts of the Soviet Union where Islam retained the strongest hold. Village mosques were officially closed, but a whole network of unofficial mullahs kept alive a very conservative brand of Islam. This was not a clandestine religion, as even Party members would summon the mullah to perform ceremonies such as circumcisions or burials. What set Tajikistan apart from the other Muslim republics was the degree to which Islam became a political issue in the wake of the collapse of the Soviet Union.

Strangely enough, given that Islam seeks to transcend differences between peoples, the driving force behind this Islamic revival was, in fact, parochialism. The districts that had been deprived of power,

The plight of Tajik refugees in Afghanistan

The refugees from Tajikistan who fled as entire kolkhozes to Afghanistan in December 1992 found themselves on arrival in an area populated by Tajiks like themselves who spoke the same language and potentially had the same enemies, the 'communists' backed by the Russians. In Afghanistan, a country at war, they were soon to become not only allies, but hostages to the various groups of Mujahideen.

Of the 60,000 refugees counted by the UNHCR, 25,000 have been regrouped in the Sakhi camp, set up near Mazar-i-Sharif, in the area controlled by General Dostam, an Uzbek and former Moscow ally turned Afghan nationalist who remains hostile to the Muslim political cause. The others are in camps in the north-east where control is in the hands of virtually independent military leaders allied to a variety of Islamic parties. Humanitarian organizations, when they tried to assist, were rapidly expelled and replaced by Muslim organizations, essentially sponsored by Saudi Arabia. The refugees were supported and trained for *jihad* by such groups, which dream of turning the town of Kunduz into another Peshawar and a base from which to win back Tajikistan and Central Asia.

The UNHCR is faced with a dilemma: either to leave the Tajik refugees in Afghanistan, risking their being dragooned into the Islamic-dominated Tajik opposition in exile, or to push them to return to Tajikistan, exposing them to the risk of harassment by the gangs of Kulyabis active in the south of the country. Between May and July 1993, several thousand refugees, mainly women and children, returned to Tajikistan, preferring uncertainty in their home country to a precarious existence in the camps, but the flow has slowed down with the revival of fighting in the border region. The Tajik refugees in Afghanistan are now political bargaining chips trapped between the dreams of revenge of the Islamic government in exile and the brutality of the government in Dushanbe.

Kurgan Tyube and the Garm Valley, rallied around Islam to oppose the regime of President Nabiyev, which had remained Soviet to the core, even after independence. The second factor that made Tajikistan so special was that the official Soviet-nominated head of the clergy, the grand Qazi Aqbar Turajanzadeh, a close associate of the Muslim Brotherhood, became leader of the Islamic opposition. In the USSR, sympathizers of the Muslim Brotherhood had set up the Islamic Renaissance Party in 1991 and its Tajik branch was one of the most active. The final factor was that the nationalist opposition (the Rastakhiz party) and the democratic opposition (the democratic party), which were restricted to the small urban intelligentsia, and the Ismailis banded together with the Islamic Renaissance Party against the communists. The Uzbek minority, meanwhile, sided with the Kulyabis and the Khojentis.

CIVIL WAR

Tajikistan was the only Central Asian republic in which an opposition coalition temporarily managed to oust the old Communist Party apparatchiks. The stand-off began in April 1992, with a demonstration by the Muslim/democratic supporters in Dushanbe, in Martyrs' Square, calling for the resignation of the president of the National Assembly. The Kulyabis demonstrated in Freedom Square, a few hundred metres away, in favour of the government. Weapons began to circulate at the beginning of May, the Kulyabis were forced to evacuate and a Muslim-democrat government was installed. It had no troops, however, apart from a few Ismaili militias. The Russian garrison, the 201st Motorized Division, remained neutral at the beginning of the crisis, but some units backed the Kulyabis when clashes began in the south of the country, in the Kurgan Tyube region. The war worsened in September, and President Nabiyev, who was still in power, was forced to step down. The Kulyabis then began to clear the south of their Muslim-democrat enemies, and they began a slow armed advance on the capital, while the 201st division became more and more open in its support of the communists. In November 1992, a parliament meeting in Khojent elected as its leader Emomali Rakhmonov, who is now head of state, and in December the Kulyab forces, supported by Uzbekistan, seized Dushanbe. This neo-communist clampdown was ferocious, with anyone from Kurgan Tyube, the Garm valley or the Pamir mountains, which were the traditional fiefs of the Muslim-democrat supporters, being struck down indiscriminately. The democrat leaders fled or were arrested, the Muslim fighters sought refuge with groups of Mujahideen in Afghanistan and the Ismailis holed up in their Pamir stronghold.

The civil war which tore the country apart for six months was extremely violent. The fighting and the massacres left approximately 50,000 dead, and 500,000 people, one-tenth of the Tajik population, took flight. The war was all the more bloody as it was based on score-settling on ethnic and parochial lines. The Ismailis in Dushanbe were massacred by the Kulyabis, who conducted manhunts in various parts of the capital, making arbitrary arrests and conducting summary executions. In the south, Kurgan Tyube was recaptured with great savagery. Entire villages were razed and their inhabitants massacred, tens of thousands of civilians were forced to take to the road and were constantly harassed by revenge-hungry armed gangs, who considered them 'enemies to be eradicated'. This is how around 60,000 people evicted from their villages came to arrive in December at the Afghan border, where they were forced, in the dead of winter, to cross the freezing waters of the Amu Darya to find refuge from their pursuers in Afghanistan. During this sombre period, humanitarian organizations never got access to Tajik territory. They were only able to bring relief in Afghanistan, but not to offer protection to people at home. The Russian border guards often fired on the refugees, but found themselves the targets when a group of refugees, armed and trained by Muslim groups in a dozen camps in north-east Afghanistan, staged a counter-attack in the spring of 1993. In July, a border post was destroyed and twenty-five border guards killed, drawing a sharp reaction from Boris Yeltsin in Moscow, who declared that the Tajik–Afghan border was 'Russia's border', and sent reinforcements to prevent further incursions. However, as the Russian army lacked volunteers prepared to die in a new 'Afghan War', it contented itself with bombing villages in the north of Afghanistan.

Clashes also continued inside Tajikistan, pitting government forces armed and backed by the Russians and Uzbeks against opposition groups entrenched in the isolated valleys to the east of Dushanbe and blocking the only route from there to the Pamirs. The 170,000 inhabitants of the Pamirs and the 60,000 who have sought refuge there since the massacres in Dushanbe are in a difficult situation. This, the 'roof of the world', depends completely on outside supplies, and since the beginning of the civil war the only humanitarian assistance has come from Kyrgyzstan, via the road skirting the Chinese border. The blockade imposed by Dushanbe and the military pressure of government forces is threatening to push the Pamiris, traditionally secular and pro-Russian in their leanings, into the arms of the Muslim fighters commanded by the Tajik Jihad Council, set up in March 1993 in Taloqan in Afghanistan.

THE RUSSIAN AND UZBEK INVOLVEMENT

Although the unrest is Tajik in origin, the background against which it has been unfolding is one of a region in constant flux. Uzbekistan, fearful of the Islamic threat, played an essential role in the return of communist rule to Tajikistan by providing weapons, air cover and even soldiers for the opponents of the 'Muslim-democrats', and it is no exaggeration to say that Tajikistan is now virtually an Uzbek protectorate.

Uzbekistan, which has a large Tajik minority, is anxious to play down the ethnic arguments and portray itself instead as the major regional power guaranteeing stability in Central Asia and Afghanistan. Uzbekistan is not seeking to alter its borders, but rather to influence its smaller neighbours and check the spread of democratic and Islamic values.

After some hesitation, Russia decided in November 1992 to back the neo-communist regimes of Central Asia, but the 201st Division did not wait for orders from Moscow to start delivering weapons and supplies to the Tajik communists. However, the Russians had no genuine plans to win back Central Asia, a particularly important factor for the large Russian population that remained there, often dating back three generations.

Fear of instability and the spectre of Islam have been joined, however, by fear of being dragged into another Afghan war. The intransigence of the government in Dushanbe, which has seemed intent on eliminating all opposition since its return to power, did not bode well for the prospects of finding a political solution to the fighting. By sending tens of thousands of refugees fleeing to Afghanistan, the government's brutal stance gave a new dimension to the problem and forced Moscow to increase further its activities on the Afghan border. In order to safeguard stability, the Russians have been relying on the Uzbeks as middlemen, and have sought to involve the republics of Central Asia more closely in protecting the border. They have also been seeking the blessing of the international community, and have asked the UN to dispatch observers.

The Tajik issue is indeed a problem for the international community, which is left wondering which international forum to turn to. The humanitarian aspect is more or less settled. The UNHCR and other aid organizations are bringing relief to the refugee camps in

Afghanistan – at least, when Islamic organizations do not prevent them from doing so – while a handful of aid groups attempt to maintain a presence among the civilians in the south of Tajikistan itself and the Pamir Mountains, where they try to make up for drastic shortages of food, fuel and medicines. But the most pressing political question today is that of the international status of Tajikistan. Officially, it is an independent state, and a member of the CIS and the CSCE, but nobody knows where it truly belongs – the CIS, Europe or the Middle East? As a 'commonwealth', the CIS is more a myth than a reality, as only Russia and Uzbekistan have shown any willingness to send troops to Tajikistan, as was demonstrated by the stillborn plan to send a Central Asian peacekeeping force there at the height of the fighting. The CSCE has little desire to assume responsibility for the Central Asian republics. The United Nations, overwhelmed by the Afghan problem and a shortage of money, set up a mission in Dushanbe in the spring of 1993, but this is little more than a symbolic presence. The international community, after assiduously ignoring the unrest in Tajikistan despite its tragic human consequences, seems to have reached the conclusion that it can do little but allow Russian intervention to proceed, on the grounds that the combination of Russian influence and a series of authoritarian governments is less worrying than the 'Islamic peril'.

The problem is made all the more intractable by the fact that behind the ideological battle lie smaller quarrels over land and power between districts, factions, clans and ethnic groups. But despite all this, it would be wrong to assume that Tajikistan's civil war is an ethnic one. The heads of the factions are all Tajik, and although Tajikistan's Uzbeks have thrown their lot in with the communists, they are not engaging in ethnic cleansing. Many Tajiks living in Uzbekistan have moreover failed to back the Muslim-democrat coalition. If anything, the crisis revolves around the Tajik identity, the very viability of Tajik nationalism, and, in short, the continued existence of an independent Tajikistan. The real threat is not that an increasingly fictional Islamic revolution will be exported, but that the country will implode.

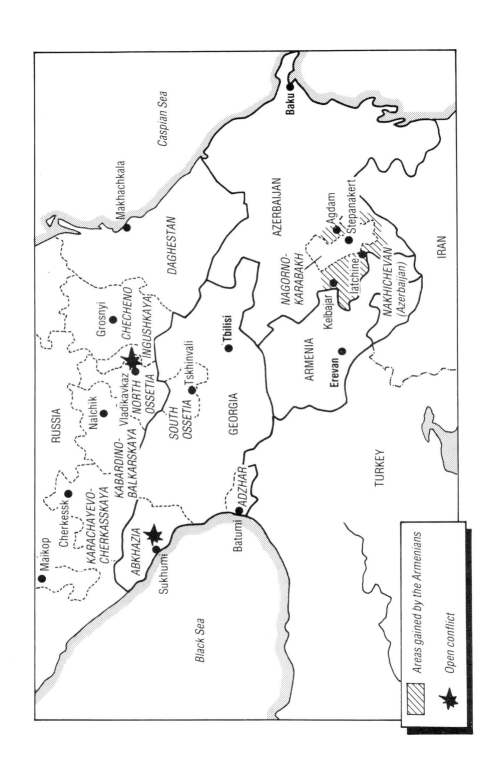

Areas gained by the Armenians

★ Open conflict

4

THE CAUCASUS
Policing the old empire

Over the last two years or so the world has focused its attention on the tragedy of Bosnia, neglecting the destruction wrought on the Caucasus by the first outbreak of inter-ethnic strife of the post-communist era, which began in 1988. Yet this was the point at which unrest was degenerating into open war, fuelled by the break-up of the Soviet army and the distribution of its weapons to the new independent states of the former Soviet Union. Since 1992, the fighting in Nagorno-Karabakh has left 10,000 dead, more than in the four preceding years taken together. In August 1992, with the fighting in South Ossetia temporarily at a standstill, war broke out first between the Abkhazians and the Georgians, and then between the Ossetians and the Ingush in the Russian-governed northern Caucasus. Moscow played a decisive role in these three conflicts, and often took sides. The former colonial power defended its actions, and asked the United Nations to recognize its troops as 'peacekeepers'. Despite many misgivings, the UN and CSCE sanctioned the *pax Russica*.

NAGORNO-KARABAKH

The hundreds of thousands of Armenians who demonstrated in 1988 for the 'reunification' of Armenia and Nagorno-Karabakh now have their wish: Armenia has to all intents and purposes seized the enclave from Azerbaijan and joined it to its territory. The price of this victory has been terrible: the war was marked by pogroms and massacres, rape and torture, with refugees streaming back and forth as the military offensives came and went and as villages were lost and won back. This continued until a single front line emerged, with the taking of the Lachin corridor in May 1992, joining the enclave to Armenia. This was the culmination of ethnic cleansing, with Armenians and Azeris in separate, ethnically uniform, areas. This did not spell the end

43

of the fighting, however. In April 1993, the Armenians expanded the corridor to the full width of the enclave by seizing the area of Kelbajar, then continued their offensives to form a cordon around Nagorno-Karabakh. The Agdam plain was occupied, looted and half-destroyed, and the Fizuli region, further south, was equally 'cleansed', resulting in the flight of hundred of thousands of civilians, who joined the scores of refugees expelled from their villages since the beginning of the fighting. The Armenians claim to have taken in 350,000 displaced persons, the Azerbaijanis 860,000, corresponding in both cases to more than 10 per cent of the population of each of the countries. Whatever the reliability of these figures, which are often inflated in the emotional climate of the region, the fact remains that hundreds of thousands of refugees and displaced persons have paid the price of a war launched on behalf of around 140,000 Armenians living in an enclave no bigger than a French *département*. This says nothing of the thousands of dead and injured, and the hundreds taken hostage on both sides. The old hatreds, which have their roots in the rivalry between the Russian Empire, the traditional 'protector' of the Armenians, and the Ottomans and the Persians in the Caucasian marches, were stifled to some degree in Soviet times, but are now resurfacing.

The West, stuck in its perception of the Armenians as 'eternal victims of the Turks', has barely stopped to wonder about their sudden victories. The latter can no doubt be attributed in part to the superior motivation and organization of the Armenians of Nagorno-Karabakh, supplied and equipped by Yerevan. What tipped the balance, however, was intelligence and logistical assistance from Moscow. Such assistance remains, as ever, largely a matter of convenience. In the years of communist 'stability', it was oil-rich Azerbaijan which tended to be favoured. In 1992, however, following Yeltsin's victory, Moscow began to support the Armenians, who had become the strongest backers of a military alliance with Russia. As it does in Tajikistan, Russia maintains an army division and a unit of border guards on the frontier with Turkey. Azerbaijan, which was governed from May 1992 to June 1993 by the nationalist and anti-Russian Popular Front, had meanwhile ordered Russian troops out. It paid the price in Nagorno-Karabakh and at home: an uprising sparked by the last Russian units in the country paved the way to the return to power in June 1993 of the ageing Geidar Aliyev, who had been Azerbaijan's leader in the Brezhnev era. Like his Georgian counterpart Shevardnadze, he had come to appear, thanks to the negligence of the nationalists, as a last-resort solution and the most popular man in the country.

Mediation efforts in Nagorno-Karabakh

When Armenia and Azerbaijan joined the United Nations in March 1992, they requested that Blue Helmets be deployed to stop the fighting in Nagorno-Karabakh. The Security Council refused to intervene, however, and left it to a regional organization, the CSCE, to try to mediate.

Nagorno-Karabakh was a test case for the CSCE, as this was the first time it had attempted to mediate in a regional dispute. In order to achieve a negotiated solution, it set in motion the 'Minsk process', which, after meetings in Rome, Prague and Geneva, was to culminate in an international peace conference. The members of the CSCE also contemplated the possibility of sending observers to supervise a ceasefire, if one could be achieved. In practice the fighting continued, the impact of diplomacy amounting to little more than visits by CSCE and UN envoys. This mediocre result demonstrated how little attention is paid to clashes which have no strategic significance and which do not threaten international borders.

Nevertheless, the spread of the fighting outside Nagorno-Karabakh was a jolt for the international community. Though the UN condemned the seizure of Lachin, it did not seek further involvement, and reiterated what it called the irreplaceable role of the CSCE process. It is impossible to tell quite how the CSCE was supposed to achieve anything given that its statutes require the politically disparate member countries to reach unanimity on every decision. While the military stand-off created another ten thousand victims, the interminable 'Minsk process' continued without results. The fall of Kelbajar and 10 per cent of Azerbaijan's territory into Armenian hands in April 1993 elicited more international response. The Security Council adopted Resolution 822, which called for an unconditional ceasefire and the withdrawal of 'expansionists' from the conquered lands. In the absence of buffer forces, however, the new Resolution has remained wishful thinking, and the fighting goes on.

Russian influence also lies at the root of a rough period for Armenia, between June and December 1992, when Moscow decided to allocate to the emerging armies of the three Trans-Caucasian republics equal quantities of arms taken from the former Soviet forces in the area, at the risk of escalating the fighting. The distribution of what was at times sophisticated weaponry, such as planes, helicopters and tanks, was in effect confirming a *status quo*, as the equipment had already been looted by local militias and, more often than not, sold off by the officers of the units stationed in the area. But this also allowed the Azerbaijanis to carry out their only successful offensive: for reasons which remain a mystery, they received their tanks a little earlier than the Armenians, and took the north of Nagorno-Karabakh, causing tens of thousands of people to flee to Stepanakert.

Dependence on the Russians also explains the lack of success of the CSCE's efforts at mediation. Moscow did not want to see them succeed until its own design for the region was in place. While the CSCE held fast to the principle of inviolability of borders, also espoused by Azerbaijan, Moscow, in order to maintain its influence in the former empire, took the side of the ethnic minorities in the 'rebel republics' seeking its support against their new 'oppressors'. As a result, the Armenians of Nagorno-Karabakh, buoyed by Moscow's backing against an Azerbaijan that had severe domestic problems and had been deserted by the Turks, rejected the CSCE's solutions, insisting that their independence be recognized first. The cowing of Azerbaijan has brought severe consequences for Armenia, though, as it is threatened with a third winter without fuel or electricity, thanks to the blockade – the losers' trump card – imposed by Baku and Ankara. The blockade has been further worsened by the fighting in Abkhazia, which has cut the last land routes linking Armenia to Russia, through Georgia.

ABKHAZIA

'Why should Georgia have the right to break free from Russia and we not have the right to secede from Georgia?'

The Abkhazians' reasoning is the same as that of most small ethnic groups in the former Soviet Union who are living in what are now independent non-Russian republics. They naturally seek Moscow's protection against the often uncompromising and fervent nationalism of these cauldrons of nationalist turmoil.

The Abkhazians had long sought to desert the Georgian camp for that of the Russians, but the Georgians, who make up 60 per cent of

Hostage dealers in Nagorno-Karabakh

Hostage-taking, an old hallmark of wars in the Caucasus, is making a comeback. In the war in Nagorno-Karabakh, the practice emerged once pogroms, rape and various forms of violence had completed the 'cleansing' of Azerbaijani and Armenian territory of the opposing ethnic group. On both sides of the front line, civilian hostages taken in fighting are traded on an *ad hoc* basis during tenuous ceasefires, as happened in July 1993 when Armenians took Baku families hostage at a wedding in a village near Fizuli. Kidnapping also occurs further from the front, as happened in the case of twenty or so Georgian Armenians taken from a Baku–Tbilisi train.

The kidnappers are not only armed gangs or ordinary families seeking the release of one of their own. Increasingly, professional 'dealers' are undertaking to facilitate the exchanges. They may be gang leaders with 'private prisons' or police or army commanders using their barracks. In the interests of easy 'business', barter may also be used, swapping one live hostage for several bodies, petrol, livestock or money – the latter preferably hard currency. The price varies, of course, according to the importance of the hostage.

The Geneva Conventions require the unconditional release of civilian prisoners, and the internment of combatants under strict control. However, neither Baku nor Yerevan have ratified these conventions, which considerably hampers the work of the ICRC. Although both republics have agreed to set up government committees to investigate the hostage problem, with which the ICRC tries to negotiate, the deadlock remains complete as Azerbaijan refuses to deal directly with the relevant commission in the self-proclaimed republic of Nagorno-Karabakh. With no settlement of this political question in sight, it is business as usual for Nagorno-Karabakh's hostage dealers.

---

the population of Abkhazia, an integral part of Georgia, were not prepared to let them go, particularly after having lost control of another of their autonomous republics, South Ossetia. This accounted for their reaction in August 1992, when they sent tanks into

Sukhumi, the capital of the Autonomous Republic of Abkhazia, which had just declared independence. This declaration seemed doomed to failure, as the Abkhazians, most of whom were driven into Turkey at the end of the last century, make up no more than 17 per cent of the republic's population. Although they had managed to ally themselves with other local minorities (Armenians, Greeks and Russians), their aim of dictating to the Georgian majority seemed unrealistic.

One year later, the Abkhazians had nevertheless succeeded in taking control of practically all of Abkhazia. This cost 2,000 lives on both sides, created 150,000 refugees and destroyed part of Sukhumi, which was still in Georgian hands and under constant bombardment. Once again, Russian support for the Abkhazians was a deciding factor, and in an even more marked way than in Azerbaijan. Backing came first and foremost from Russian nationalists and communists, who had made the fate of the former USSR's minorities and Russian-speakers their hobby-horse, but Moscow rapidly took up the cause, describing it in more elegant terms as defending the rights of minorities to autonomy within republics whose own territorial integrity was assured. Another factor was the support of the Russian military, who attached great importance to an alliance with an autonomous Abkhazia to provide them with more access to the Black Sea, after the loss of the Crimea and Odessa, now part of Ukraine. Russian involvement in the fighting forced a weakened Georgia to sign a ceasefire agreement in July 1993. The Georgians then had to agree to withdraw their troops from Abkhazia and to grant it autonomy, guaranteed by forces which were largely composed of Russian troops and not an international force, as Tbilisi had wished. The UN limited itself to sending fifty observers to enforce the ceasefire under conditions determined by Moscow. This was an approach modelled on that used to resolve the conflict between the South Ossetians and the Georgians, which, like the fighting in Moldavia, was brought to a halt in 1992 by the intervention of Russian forces dressed up as 'joint buffer forces' by the addition of a few Ossetians and Georgians, and later by CSCE military observers. But the ceasefire was violated by the Abkhazians in September, and the fall of Sukhumi worsened the fears of Georgians, haunted by the idea of disappearing as a nation.

THE NORTHERN CAUCASUS

On the northern slopes of the Caucasus, within the Russian Federation, live a dozen small and mostly Muslim ethnic groups who also hope one day to achieve independence. They are descendants of the mountain-dwellers who fought long 'holy wars' against the armies of the Tsar in the nineteenth century. Some were deported to Central Asia in 1944 under the pretext that they had collaborated with the Nazis; this was Stalin's solution to their obstinate refusal to toe the line. The survivors were able to return under Khrushchev, but one of these 'exiled peoples', the Ingush, found some of what had been their land occupied by the North Ossetians, close relatives of the South Ossetians and traditionally loyal to Moscow.

In November 1992, the serious tension between the Ingush and the Ossetians degenerated into extremely violent confrontation to the east of Vladikavkaz, where some 60,000 Ingush had managed to resettle themselves on their old lands, among Ossetians and Cossacks. Russian troops intervened, allegedly as a buffer force but they openly and brutally sided with the Ossetians and attacked Ingush villages with tank fire, causing hundreds of deaths. The survivors were driven out to what was left of their territory, a rump republic attached to that of their Chechen cousins, which is alone in having asserted independence – though Moscow has no intention of recognizing this – by expelling Russian troops. The Ingush, encouraged by the Chechen, continue to lay claim to their land. There is constant confrontation in this highly unstable part of Russia's southern confines, where Moscow is upholding a state of emergency buttressed by large numbers of troops.

THE RUSSIAN DESIGN

The resurgence of Moscow's activism in Trans-Caucasia is partly explained by its desire to retain control of the area bordering the southern flank – and 'weak link' – of the Russian Federation, where the Muslim population is a focus of attention for Turkey and even Iran. Russia has found fertile ground here because of the presence of minorities seeking its support. The avowed aim is to make Georgia and Azerbaijan – coincidentally the only republics outside the CIS – into federations modelled on Russia.

The United States, the EC and NATO have been content to watch Russia intervene in conflicts which are too complicated and too far removed from their direct spheres of interest for them to hope to exert any real influence, even supposing that they had any such intention after their dithering in what was Yugoslavia. When Boris Yeltsin appealed to the international community at the beginning of 1993 to provide funding for Russian intervention in conflicts in the former USSR, the response was lukewarm. The treatment of the Ingush minority in the Russian Federation made it difficult for Moscow to argue convincingly that its action in other republics was designed only to defend the rights of minorities. The inability of the United Nations to become involved in these clashes amounted, however, to the international community's sanctioning of Moscow's arbitrary policing of its former empire.

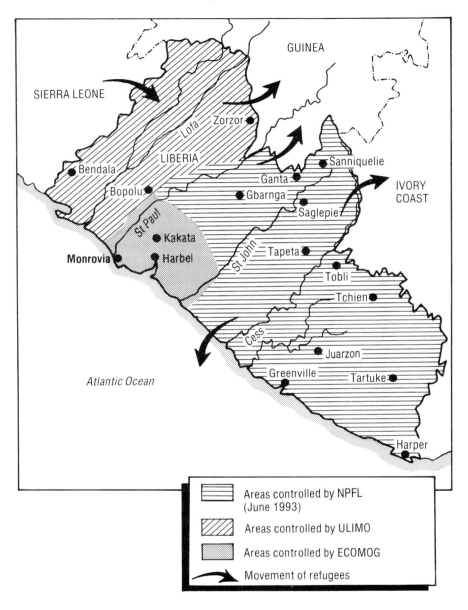

Areas controlled by NPFL (June 1993)	
Areas controlled by ULIMO	
Areas controlled by ECOMOG	
Movement of refugees	

5

LIBERIA
Leave it to the neighbours

Long before Somalia, Liberia was the first African country to commit
'national suicide'. It has been ravaged since December 1989 by fighting of extreme cruelty, the initial phase of which drove out nearly
700,000 refugees. However, the massacres and atrocities were not
enough to reverse the indifference of the international community or
to provoke a significant reaction from the United States, despite its
close involvement with Liberia since the foundation of the country. In
the absence of UN action, with the political and financial support of
the international community, the countries of West Africa have been
trying since the summer of 1990 to manage this troublespot. This, the
first regional peacekeeping initiative in an African country, certainly
put an end to the massacres among ethnic groups in the capital, but
it compromised itself by its involvement with armed groups responsible for atrocities and ended up by becoming a participant in the
conflict.

THE DESCENT INTO CHAOS

Fighting in Liberia started on 24 December 1989 with the incursion of
a force of about fifty National Patriotic Front of Liberia (NPFL) rebels
from the Ivory Coast. The first battles were followed by bloody
reprisals by Samuel Doe's government troops, resulting in a mass
exodus. Within a few months, hundreds of thousands had taken
refuge in Guinea and the Ivory Coast in camps which soon became
base camps and a recruitment centre for the NPFL. Meanwhile, in
Liberia itself, the rebels made rapid progress towards Monrovia and
surrounded the town in July 1990. In spite of the violence of the
fighting and the scale of the atrocities, the conflict provoked no
reaction from the international community: the United States merely
stationed warships offshore from the capital, protected its embassy

and evacuated its citizens; the United Nations, anxious not to become directly involved, looked for a regional proxy and backed the initiatives of the Economic Community of West African States (ECOWAS). In August 1990, ECOWAS deployed its Ceasefire Monitoring Group (ECOMOG) in Monrovia, which was also mandated to establish an interim government. The 'White Helmets', landing in a devastated capital, empty of diplomats and with only a handful of relief organizations attempting to carry on under appalling conditions, stopped the rebels' advance, depriving them *in extremis* of their final victory. In a besieged Monrovia, crowded with refugees from all over Liberia, living in fear of a final tribal score-settling, there was a general sense of relief. However, left without a sufficiently clear mandate, the regional peacekeeping force could not provide a solution to either the political causes or the disastrous humanitarian consequences of the conflict.

In November 1990, following three months of skirmishes between soldiers of the West African force and NPFL fighters, a precarious truce was established on both sides of the 'front line', a vague no-man's-land surrounding the capital. The truce held for nearly two years until October 1992, in spite of numerous incidents. Throughout this period, the regional peacekeeping force occupied the capital where an 'interim government of national unity', led by Professor Amos Sawyer, was set up with its support. However, Charles Taylor's NPFL controlled 90 per cent of Liberia. Following painstaking negotiations between the increasingly numerous Liberian factions and hard bargaining between ECOWAS member states, ever more divided over the objectives of their action, the 'Yamoussoukro IV agreement' was signed in October 1991 in the political capital of the Ivory Coast. It provided for ECOMOG to be deployed throughout the country, armed forces to be confined to camp and multi-party elections to be held at the end of a one-year transitional period.

However, the fragile hopes for peace were finally buried by the arrival from neighbouring Sierra Leone of a new armed faction, the United Liberation Movement of Liberia for Democracy (ULIMO), made up of former soldiers of Samuel Doe and exiles fiercely hostile to Charles Taylor. ULIMO dislodged the NPFL from the west of the country, provoking a massive NPFL attack on Monrovia in October 1992. Thus Charles Taylor ended the process of normalization, denouncing ULIMO as the 'ECOMOG death squad'. Faced with a resurgence of fighting, ECOMOG went on the offensive, pounding coastal towns with its warships and carrying out numerous air attacks on the territory controlled by the NPFL, which was also subjected to an economic blockade. The resurgence of fighting further disrupted

Humanitarian aid in the line of fire

In Saniquellie, northern Liberia, on 18 April 1993, two ECOMOG Alpha jets attacked a convoy heading for Ganta. For several weeks the peacekeeping force had been carrying out air raids on territory controlled by the NPFL. However, the target was far from being a military target: the trucks were clearly marked with the MSF symbol. And MSF was not there illegally: according to ECOWAS rules and Security Council Resolution 813, the embargo imposed a few months earlier on NPFL territory does not apply to humanitarian aid; on the contrary, it is part of the White Helmets' task to protect it.

A complaint was sent to the ECOWAS Presidency and requests for support were sent to the UN and the EC. Their first reactions came in the form of a few polite letters of support followed, a few days later, by decisions that were to bear serious consequences.

ECOWAS unilaterally announced the closure of the border with the Ivory Coast and the opening of a new corridor, which it christened the 'peace corridor' – a nice euphemism, considering it is supposed to cross the front line and is therefore totally impassable. NPFL territory was thus encircled and a total block-ade imposed. Unable to restore peace thus far, ECOMOG decided to impose it by any means and was prepared to break a few principles in the name of a speedy solution. The diplomats acquiesced, the politicians gave their consent and all agreed that the Liberian mess called for a big clean-up operation. The UN Secretary-General's special envoy put it bluntly: 'Certain organ-izations have the task of bringing relief to those in need. We have a more important task: bringing peace. If relief gets in the way of peacemaking then there will be no relief.'

Carte blanche? It certainly means that the logic of war takes over completely: the only solution would be the disappearance of one of the warring factions. And so much the better if that enables the United Nations to avoid getting caught up in Liberia. For who is better placed to resolve a regional conflict than a regional force?

a society already torn apart during the first months of the conflict: nearly a quarter of the country's population was forced to remain in wretched exile in neighbouring countries and, inside the country, the shortages resulting from the blockade, the air raids and the continuous shifting of the front line forced tens of thousands to flee their homes, and led to starvation and epidemics.

This third phase of the conflict, which started with the arrival on the scene of ULIMO and ended in general war-weariness in the summer of 1993, seems to have convinced all the belligerents that a 'final victory' was impossible, and to have renewed hopes for a negotiated settlement. In July 1993, all the factions accepted a new ceasefire and a detailed timetable for transition. For the first time the United Nations became politically involved, deploying observers to monitor the ceasefire. The faction leaders agreed in principle to disarm their forces and confine them to camp, but it remains uncertain whether these undertakings will be honoured: Charles Taylor made similar commitments following the Yamoussoukro agreement but soon renounced them, claiming that 'his hand had been forced'. Only time will tell whether this latest cessation of hostilities marks the beginning of a solution or a momentary lull in the fighting.

Charles Taylor does need a respite. The NPFL ended a two-year break in the fighting in October 1992, when it launched an all-out offensive, throwing all its forces into the battle to take the capital, Monrovia. During the often suicidal-looking 'Operation Octopus', as it was called, Charles Taylor's supporters, fighting fiercely around Monrovia and in the suburbs, forced more than 200,000 people to flee to the town centre. Another aspect of the war was the suicidal bravery in street-fighting of the NPFL Small Boys Unit, a special unit put together out of young orphans brutally conditioned by the war. Once again, as at the very beginning of the conflict, Charles Taylor's fighters transformed the 'liberation war' into a 'carnival of blood' during their victorious march on the capital. Constantly drunk or high on marijuana, wearing wigs, wedding dresses or welder's goggles, they acted out the profound identity crisis into which their shattered world has plunged them. This 'deviant' behaviour, displayed in varying degrees by all the factions, has roots that must be far more complex than that 'tribal war' that has often been called responsible. The five European ambassadors, meeting one last time in Monrovia before their evacuation from the country, termed the nascent chaos 'national suicide', in a reference to Liberia's bloody history. Whatever explanations are put forward, the extreme cruelty of the Liberian conflict reflects the country's recent past.

THE LIBERIAN RIFT

Well before the start of the present war, which is civil only in terms of its victims, the history of Liberia was punctuated with bloodbaths. The massacres started in 1980 when Samuel Doe took power, ending 133 years of Afro-American hegemony in this country founded in 1847 by former American slaves. The 'master sergeants' coup', which resulted in President Tolbert's assassination and then the execution of the governing elite on Monrovia beach, was welcomed by the Liberian 'natives' as the final revenge for the 'black-on-black' colonial-style oppression. The excesses of this bloody 'decolonization' soon became common practice and in 1983, and again in 1985, the army commander, Brigadier-General Thomas Quiwonkpa, tried unsuccessfully to prevent the repressive zeal of the new government. After the failure of the second attempted coup, the army launched a punitive expedition into the rebels' tribal lands, home of the Gio and Mano peoples in north-eastern Liberia. Bloody retribution was visited upon the region, feeding a lasting hatred of the government. In December 1989 it took just a few dozen trained men crossing the border with neighbouring Ivory Coast to provoke an immediate insurrection, especially as the Armed Forces of Liberia (AFL), made up essentially of Krahn, President Samuel Doe's ethnic group, had carried out a new wave of indiscriminate tribal reprisals. With the rebels at the gates of the capital, the hard-pressed government army pitilessly pursued the Gio and Mano in Monrovia. On the night of 29 July 1990, some 600 civilians, including many women and children, who had taken refuge in Saint Paul's church under the protection of the Red Cross, were massacred in cold blood. Not to be outdone, the NPFL executed or butchered members of the Krahn ethnic group and also of the Mandingo, Muslim merchants accused of 'collusion' with Samuel Doe's Government. Deprived of their victory when they had all but entered Monrovia, the rebels set about looting and terrorizing the territory under their control. Mass graves, some containing hundreds of bodies, were discovered all round the Liberian capital following the retreat of the NPFL.

None of the Liberian factions escaped this cycle of terror, which carried thousands of people into a dizzy spiral of violence and atrocities. None of them tried to limit the looting and massacres perpetrated by their 'fighters', let alone punish those responsible. Right up to its formal dissolution at the end of 1992, Prince Johnson's Independent National Patriotic Front of Liberia (INPFL) acted with the same cruelty as the original rebel movement. ULIMO, recruiting among former AFL soldiers, inherited the methods of the former 'national' army. Even the interim government of Professor Amos Sawyer has blood on its hands, although to a lesser degree: its 'black berets', a militia force of some 500 men, is in practice an integral part of what remains of the former government army. Fighting often side by side with ECOMOG, which has no unified command structure but coordinates its actions in the field with these 'back-up troops', the AFL and ULIMO were guilty of frequent brutality and human rights violations. ECOMOG is also responsible for abuses, if not war crimes, particularly since its mandate has been interpreted as covering peacemaking by direct military engagement with Charles Taylor's troops. Apart from looting and numerous arbitrary arrests followed by violent interrogations, the West African force is responsible for murderous air attacks resulting in many civilian casualties. ECOMOG attempted to obtain a military victory by imposing a blockade and carrying out bombing raids that brought them into conflict with the relief organizations trying to bring aid to those in need without discrimination. This policy brought them under suspicion and they were accused of prolonging the conflict by providing assistance to rebel-held areas. Hospitals were bombed on a number of occasions and relief convoys, clearly identified as such, were attacked by the Nigerian air force, which sought to prevent all access to territory controlled by the NPFL. The United Nations, in the person of the Secretary-General's special envoy, backed this position, much to the annoyance of the UN agencies, which urged that aid operations should continue. It took vigorous protests from the relief organizations for the principle of free access to victims to be reaffirmed in the new agreement of July 1993.

The brutality of the Liberian conflict poses questions about the underlying causes of such remorseless violence, which appears to be both the root cause and the result of the emergence of a new breed of political adventurer. Such people have 'criminalized' the whole country so that it operates on the basis of war and predatory instinct alone. In this context, humanitarian aid is either impossible, as a result of the literally 'insane' state of insecurity, or manipulated and looted by the armed factions, or blocked by the very people who should be protecting it. In any case, providing aid is always difficult, due to the lack of reliable partners and the systematic violation of the most elementary rules of human dignity.

The Liberian conflict also raises the issue of regional intervention as a substitute for or alternative to international action. In addition to the geopolitical marginalization of the African continent and the West's lack of interest in the conflict, there is a fear that material considerations partly explain the option of regional 'subcontracting': over a thirty-month period, the deployment of ECOMOG cost a third as much as the budget allocated by the United Nations to its Somalia operation for the last eight months of 1993. At a time when an increasing number of peacekeeping operations require ever greater financial support from ever more reluctant countries, it is easier to understand the arguments put forward by Edward Perkins, US Ambassador to the United Nations: speaking to the Security Council on 18 November 1992, he justified his support for a regional solution by saying that if the concerted ECOWAS effort in Liberia failed, ECOWAS would probably withdraw from peacekeeping and the resolution of regional conflicts, which would increase the pressure on the UN and the United States to take direct action. Nevertheless, this kind of regional action, which has become so popular with the international community, is not without its problems: while there is no denying that the West African force 'contained' the Liberian tragedy, it is clear that political motives were not absent from the decision of the regional power, Nigeria, to lead the task force that rapidly became one of the parties to the conflict. Anxious to avoid any involvement in Liberia, the international community supported the ECOMOG action politically and financially, at the risk of endorsing and sanctioning its reprehensible practices and the questionable directions it has taken.

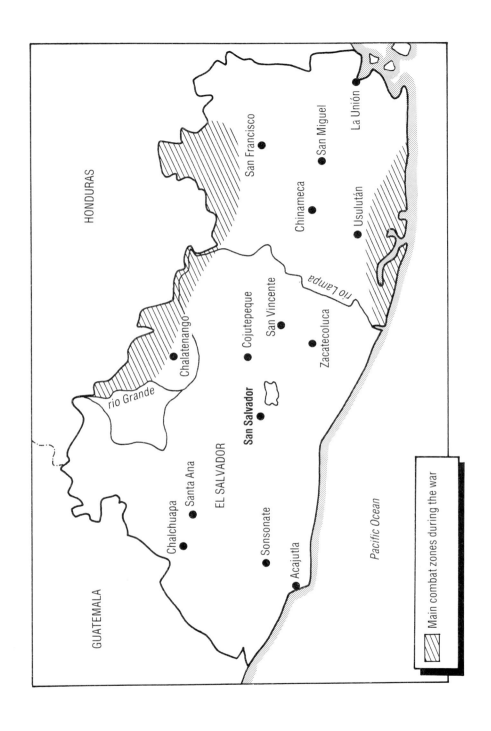

HONDURAS

San Francisco

San Miguel

La Unión

Chinameca

Usulután

rio Lampa

GUATEMALA

Chalatenango

rio Grande

Cojutepeque

San Vincente

Zacatecoluca

Santa Ana

San Salvador

EL SALVADOR

Chalchuapa

Sonsonate

Acajutla

Pacific Ocean

Main combat zones during the war

6

EL SALVADOR
The guarantor of peace

On 1 February 1992 the guns at last fell silent in El Salvador, after twelve years of civil war that had claimed 80,000 lives, most of them civilians, and seen large numbers of the population subjected to repression. The Chapultepec peace agreements formally ended the conflict that had pitted the marxist guerrilla movement Frente Farabundo Marti para la Liberacion Nacional (FMLN) against the US-backed government. Social injustice and the lack of democracy lay at the root of a civil war that was nurtured by the East–West conflict: with the end of the Cold War, a negotiated settlement became possible. From the outset, the United Nations acted as mediator and guarantor in the negotiating process – a role that went well beyond mere peacekeeping – helping to restore confidence and encourage the search for a political solution.

TWELVE YEARS OF WAR

The spark that ignited El Salvador's civil war was the *coup d'état* mounted by a group of young, reform-oriented officers, who in October 1979 overthrew the government headed by General Humberto Romero, last in a long line of iron-fisted patricians who had ruled El Salvador on behalf of the big landowners ever since the crushing of the peasants' revolt of 1932. The *coup d'état* and the war it heralded were a reaction to the political and social turmoil of the previous decade. Tensions had been mounting throughout the 1970s, and the shortage of land was further exacerbated by the return of 100,000 Salvadorean peasants expelled by Honduras after a clash between the two countries. With 212 inhabitants per square kilometre (six times the regional average), El Salvador is an overpopulated country where the coffee bean is king, and where the best land has traditionally been disproportionately concentrated in the hands of a small number of large landowners, 40 per cent of the land suitable for cultivation being owned by 0.5 per cent of the population.

Guerrilla groups were formed and a powerful popular movement sprang up, taking to the streets to demand change. The government responded with repression, blocking any chance of political liberalization by imposing its own stooges in three rigged elections in ten years. The initiators of the 1979 *coup* raised new hopes by appointing civilians to the government, but their reforming zeal came to nothing. Egged on by the oligarchy, the army hardliners maintained their repressive stance and blocked the junta's initiatives, especially where agrarian reform was concerned, thus prompting the resignation of civilian moderates.

The war between the US-backed regime and the guerrilla movement supported by the communist world, in particular the USSR, East Germany, Nicaragua and Cuba, went through a number of phases. On the political front, the Christian Democrat Napoleon Duarte governed virtually without interruption from 1984 to 1989, presiding over a democratization process from which the left was excluded, while his tentative overtures towards the FMLN were frustrated by extremists on both sides.

However, the victory of the ARENA (Alianza Republicana Nacional) candidate in the presidential elections of 1989 ironically paved the way for a negotiated settlement: businessman Alfredo Cristiani represented the pragmatic movement emerging within ARENA, originally a party of the far right that had long been dominated by the figure of Major d'Abuisson, who was accused of being behind the assassination of the Archbishop of San Salvador, Monsignor Romero, in 1980.

On the military front, after the failure of its 'all-out offensive' in 1981, the guerrilla movement was pushed back into the countryside. In spite of numerous offensives launched by an army equipped and advised by the United States, it remained unvanquished until 1986, when it again began to make its presence felt in the towns and cities. Towards the end of 1989 it rocked the government to the core with a large-scale attack on the capital itself.

THE HIGHEST CIVILIAN TOLL

The civilian population was devastated by the conflict, which claimed 80,000 lives and created tens of thousands of invalids, widows and orphans and more than a million refugees and displaced persons. The first three years of the war were marked by a veritable reign of terror. The security forces and the 'death squads' (military or paramilitary

Human rights in the service of peace

The Truth Commission's report on human rights violations, published on 15 March 1993 under the auspices of the United Nations, was one of the turning points in the peace process. The conclusions of the three-member Commission were a particularly damning indictment of the Salvadorean military's top brass.

A team of international lawyers heard the testimony of 2,000 witnesses and processed information on some 20,000 acts of violence. The report placed the blame for at least 6,200 human rights violations squarely on the shoulders of the security forces, and found the guerrilla forces guilty of a further 800 such violations.

The Commission recommended the dismissal of 400 officers, including the Minister of Defence and his deputy, together with that of fourteen Supreme Court judges accused of covering up atrocities. The report also requested that fifteen FMLN officials, including one of its five leaders, be barred from holding public office.

Among the worst crimes, the report cited the assassination of Archbishop Oscar Romero by a 'death squad' in 1980; the murder of four American nuns by the national guard in 1980; the slaughter of several hundred peasants by the army's elite battalions, in particular the River Sumpul (1980) and El Mozote (1981) massacres; and the murder of six Jesuit priests, their employee and his daughter in 1989, on orders issued by the high command.

The report also condemned an FMLN faction for the murder of civilians, the execution of eleven mayors between 1985 and 1988, and the carnage of Zona Rosa, where four US soldiers and nine civilians died on a restaurant terrace.

Just five days after the report was published, the National Assembly, dominated by the ARENA party, approved a general amnesty proposed by President Cristiani, a decision that was roundly condemned both in El Salvador and abroad, and which prompted the United States to suspend military aid. However, even though not a single soldier, death squad member or guerrilla fighter will have to face a tribunal, virtually all the army's high command was dismissed.

personnel operating out of uniform) kidnapped, tortured and killed anyone suspected of sympathizing with the 'subversives', murdering 13,000 civilians in 1980 and as many again the following year. Meanwhile, out in the country, the army was slaughtering peasants by the hundred.

The repression subsequently became more selective, targeting political activists, trade unionists, students and human rights activists. Equipped by the US with a powerful air force, the military carried out large-scale bombing campaigns to drive the local population out of areas in which the FMLN was active. However, the armed forces did not have a monopoly in human rights violations: the guerrillas also executed local officials, prisoners, ARENA members and enemy 'informers', and indulged in bloodthirsty internal score-settling. Conscription and the indiscriminate use of antipersonnel mines were common practice.

The presence of the international media, American public opinion and the government's espousal of democratic values were undoubtedly responsible for the scaling down of the conflict after the black years of 1979–82, and these factors made it easier to get humanitarian aid in. In spite of the violence, humanitarian organizations went on operating in the war zones throughout the conflict, with the consent of both parties, and it was generally possible to get help to victims of the fighting. Although both sides on occasion sought to obstruct aid operations, they at least refrained from making them into targets.

The peace process got under way in the months following the FMLN's San Salvador offensive, an operation that finally dashed all government hopes of a military victory just as the collapse of state socialism and the electoral defeat of the Sandinistas in Nicaragua deprived the guerrillas of their outside backing. The end of the Cold War also forced the government and the Salvadorean establishment to seek a compromise: they knew they could no longer count on handouts from the US and realized that a military solution was out of the question. The United States too, less paranoid about the 'communist threat' in the new international environment, urged the generals to negotiate.

A POSITIVE INTERNATIONAL INVOLVEMENT

The new climate that brought the two sides to the negotiating table also allowed the United Nations to become involved in the peace process, first just as observers, then as active mediators – to the extent of drafting part of the final treaty – and ultimately as guarantors of compliance with that treaty on the ground.

The participation of the international community undoubtedly contributed to the success of the negotiations, which would in all probability have broken down at some stage between the convening of the Geneva talks (April 1990) and the signing of the agreements in Chapultepec, Mexico (January 1992) had it not been for the commitment of UN Secretary-General Javier Perez de Cuellar, pressure from Washington and the good offices of Spain, Costa Rica, Venezuela and Colombia. The Catholic Church, which had always sought to promote dialogue, was also closely involved in the peace process.

In July 1990 the government and the FMLN signed the San José agreement on human rights, thus drawing a line under the abuses of the ten-year conflict. The two parties asked the UN to take all necessary measures to promote and defend human rights, authorizing it to speak to anyone it pleased, to go anywhere it wished in El Salvador and to visit any place or establishment without prior notice, including barracks and prisons.

HUMAN RIGHTS AT THE HUB OF THE PEACE PROCESS

This agreement had the virtue of placing the issue of human rights, which had to a certain extent been the cause of the conflict in the first place, very much at the hub of the peace process. The government's willingness to place itself in the United Nations' hands on such a sensitive issue as human rights monitoring and the investigation of violations is certainly a first in the history of the modern world. The presence of the Blue Helmets of the UN Observer Mission in El Salvador (ONUSAL), which were deployed from July 1991 – i.e., before the conclusion of the negotiations – in rural areas and war zones, kept the lid on the fighting in general and violence to the civilian population in particular.

The people of El Salvador waited for the ceasefire to enter into force, which it duly did on 1 February 1992, before celebrating this unlooked-for conclusion to the negotiations. The guerrilla movement agreed to stand down its combat units, destroy its weapons and turn itself into a legal party within nine months. The FMLN drew the line at having its men join the army, but under the agreement the military was obliged to reduce its forces by half, disband its elite units and dismiss officers guilty of human rights violations. The enforcement squads were also broken up, and the policing of law and order entrusted to a new civilian force that incorporated soldiers and former guerrillas.

The government also undertook to recognize the title of peasants to land they had occupied in guerrilla-held areas and to give plots of land to the former FMLN fighters. Finally, the electoral and legal reforms negotiated in 1991 were ratified by the national assembly.

PIONEERING ROLE FOR ONUSAL

Following the signing of the agreements, the UN Security Council approved a broader role for ONUSAL: the United Nations would supervise observance of the ceasefire and the separation of the two sides, maintaining law and order until the civilian police force was in a position to take over. The hundred or so members of the human rights division (observers, instructors, lawyers and military and police personnel) were joined by a 360-strong military division and a 230-strong police force.

Two other bodies were set up by the treaty: an 'Ad Hoc Commission' made up of three Salvadorean independents whose brief was to identify military personnel guilty of corruption, incompetence or human rights violations, and a 'Truth Commission' made up of three non-Salvadoreans appointed by the UN Secretary-General to apportion the blame for the major crimes committed during the war.

The war was officially declared at an end more than two months behind schedule, in December 1992, when the FMLN demobilized the last of its 8,000-strong force. To bring this about, the ONUSAL staff had to go well beyond their original mandate, interpreting sometimes hazy or incomplete agreements, arbitrating in disputes and on occasion demanding commitments and concessions from both sides. However, this extension of the mandate required UN officials to take on complex tasks for which they were not prepared, such as the crucial problem of land distribution and the reintegration of former guerrillas, soldiers and invalids.

To inject fresh momentum after progress had ground to a halt in April 1992, ONUSAL even went as far as to publish assessments of each side's attitude. Most of the blame lay with the government, which instead of disbanding the enforcement squads integrated them into the army, and which had fallen behind in the distribution of land. For its part, the FMLN had encouraged its supporters to occupy properties illegally, and was suspected of having hidden some of its weapons from the UN inspectors; evidence that came to light a year later proved that this was indeed the case.

A second serious crisis arose at the beginning of 1993, requiring the intervention of the new UN Secretary-General, Boutros Boutros-Ghali, who on 7 January asked President Cristiani to comply with the peace agreements by dismissing certain officers. It must be said that the 'Ad Hoc Commission' had caused something of a stir by recommending the dismissal of virtually the entire army high command.

International pressure finally overcame the military chiefs' posturing and on 30 June the Minister of Defence himself was among the last fifteen senior officers to be 'retired' by the President. In the meantime, the 'Truth Commission' had identified them as the main culprits responsible for the crimes of the previous decade.

The UN team met further obstacles which it attempted to tackle in mid-1993. Owing to the lack of official backing, the new police force and the office of the public prosecutor for human rights were several months late in getting off the ground. It was only thanks to outside assistance that these two institutions – of such vital importance to the security of former guerrilla fighters as the army, even in its reduced, purged state, is still commanded by officers trained in the school of civil war – were able to begin work under extremely difficult conditions. Furthermore, the legal system that had condoned the worst atrocities during the conflict remained in place, and the ultra-conservative judiciary, whose role was not addressed in the peace agreements, remained reluctant to collaborate with ONUSAL lawyers.

A SUCCESSFUL INTERVENTION

Even if the UN was helped by the new international climate and the willingness of President Cristiani and the FMLN to commit themselves to finding a negotiated settlement, its contribution was decisive, allowing the ceasefire to come into force, supervising the disarmament process and expediting the purging of the armed forces. During the crucial period when, despite the shared desire to find a political solution to the conflict, the gulf created between the two sides by twelve years of fighting was far from being bridged, there can be no question that the UN's role as arbitrator and guarantor helped establish a certain degree of trust between government and guerrillas and marginalized the extremists in both camps.

However, in spite of this success, the situation remains volatile and the coming months will show if the democratic progress provided for in the treaty, and into which ONUSAL has enthusiastically tried to breathe life, can survive the departure of the UN team.

The first significant pointer will be the elections scheduled for

March 1994, in which the FMLN will participate in its new guise as a social-democratic party: an open campaign followed by a fair and free vote will be the best proof of El Salvador's conversion to democratic ways and of the beneficial influence of the international community.

Beyond the elections, the role of the civilian police force and the human rights and justice departments will also be crucial. Social inequality has not been eradicated, the agrarian reforms remain incomplete and 220,000 peasant farmers are still without land. New tensions will undoubtedly arise to put Salvadorean society to the test. Only then will we know if ONUSAL has managed to instil a new political culture, or if all its efforts will have amounted to no more than a hiatus in the cruel and violent history of El Salvador.

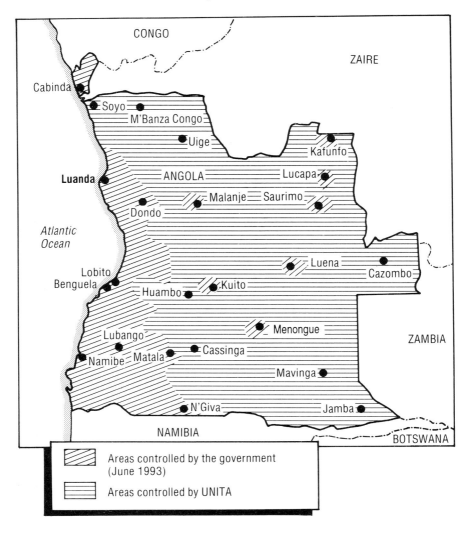

Areas controlled by the government
(June 1993)

Areas controlled by UNITA

7

ANGOLA
Stewarding the ballot box, not the peace

After a brief respite Angola is again racked by war. The fighting between the UNITA opposition and the governing MPLA, which started when the country became independent, was brought to an end by a peace agreement in May 1991. But the period of calm did not last long: the 'peace and democratization process' organized by the international community broke down in the face of UNITA's refusal to recognize the results of the September 1992 elections, even though they were pronounced 'free and fair' by the UN. So, after an interlude of a year and a half, the war goes on, more violent and bloody than before, marking a humiliating setback for the international community.

COLD WAR AND NATIONAL DIVISIONS

The struggle between UNITA and the MPLA predated independence and had its roots in the divisions of the nationalist movement. When Angola became independent in 1975 the conflict degenerated into a bloody civil war with Cuban troops, supported by the USSR, fighting on the side of the MPLA, and the South African army, backed by the US, fighting on the side of UNITA. The MPLA's victory made Angola a pawn in the Cold War and only when East–West tension lessened was it possible to get agreement, in New York in December 1988, on the withdrawal of Cuban troops, Namibian independence and an end to South African support for UNITA.

But the war continued with the US and the USSR still pulling the strings until the MPLA was forced to enter into negotiations that led to the signing of the Bicesse agreements in May 1991.

This sixteen-year-long war, in which both sides received large amounts of aid and weaponry, has left hundreds of thousands dead and tens of thousands disabled, and caused huge population movements: more than 350,000 Angolans are refugees in neighbouring

71

countries and millions have fled to the towns where they eke out a precarious existence and try to escape conscription into the army. The war has virtually paralysed production, apart from oil extraction, and made farming impossible in a countryside devastated by war, riddled with mines and mostly out of the reach of international aid.

The belligerents have also been badly scarred by the war. Behind its Marxist-Leninist rhetoric and authoritarian approach, the MPLA, fat on oil revenues, has become a corrupt *nomenklatura* out of touch with people's needs. UNITA has become increasingly militarized and is now an implacable war machine designed to crush all opposition in its path.

THE WRONG KIND OF PEACE

Each side had its own reasons to sign the agreements, which had nothing to do with the country's desire for peace and reconciliation: the MPLA signed because it had no choice and UNITA because it was convinced that the MPLA's tarnished image and the conditions laid down in the agreements made election victory a foregone conclusion. The Bicesse agreements were brokered by a troika made up of the old colonial power, Portugal, and the war's two 'godfathers', the US and the USSR. Although the stated aim was multi-party elections, the nature of the agreements precluded any chance of real democracy – 'non-belligerent Angolans' were given no say during the transition period, reinforcing the polarization of Angola and making 'democracy' the exclusive property of the two warring parties. The MPLA and UNITA shared power in the run-up to the elections, answerable only to each other and free of any constraints from the rest of Angolan society.

In addition to the lack of any grassroots controls, there was a failure, despite the troika's involvement, to provide for international monitoring of the agreements' implementation during the transition process, a task that would have been incumbent upon the UN. Called in at the last moment to give the agreements its blessing and help implement them, the UN found itself working in a subordinate role with paltry resources. Its work was subject to decisions by the Joint Political–Military Commission, on which it sat only 'by invitation'. Moreover, its mandate was extremely restrictive: it could only 'observe', not run, the elections, the organization of which remained in the hands of the government. Even on matters over which it did have authority – crucial matters such as police neutrality, enforcement of the ceasefire, organizing assembly areas, and the demobilizing and

The UN's Special Relief Programme: the failure of aid corridors

In 1990 the UN set up a special emergency aid programme for Angola, the SRPA. The aim was to bring relief to some two million victims of the civil war by creating 'corridors of peace' to provide regular access to areas cut off by the fighting. Implementation of the programme called for close coordination between NGOs, the government and UN agencies.

In practice, however, improved coordination between UN agencies has been confined to the setting-up of an additional body with a staff of 200. NGOs have been virtually ignored, despite their long experience in delivering aid throughout the Angolan war. They are treated as mere subcontractors.

The programme was modelled on Sudan's Operation Lifeline, and was an early example of an 'off-the-shelf' aid package. But because it was not tailored to the specific situation in Angola, it quickly ran into trouble. The UN's inflexibility, combined with an obligation to work in close cooperation with the national authorities precluded quick adjustments to a constantly changing situation.

But the main stumbling block was the condition that implementation required the agreement of both parties. Although the SRPA was unveiled in March 1990, it did not get under way until December, only to be suspended almost immediately until March the following year: even then only one-tenth of the programmed aid was actually distributed. Food aid became a key bargaining chip that was used ruthlessly by the warring sides with the result that the planned regular flow of aid was reduced to an occasional trickle that escaped the UN agencies' control. Often aid convoys with all the right authorizations were cancelled, held up by mines or even attacked.

In fact the corridors functioned normally only for the brief interlude between the signing of the peace agreements in June 1991 and the resumption of hostilities in September 1992. The renewed fighting meant that most people in the war zones were again cut off from aid supplies. Sadly, Angola provides but a further illustration of the failure of the very concept of 'aid corridors'.

disarming of the two armies – it was subordinate to joint MPLA–UNITA supervisory structures that had direct authority.

To cap it all, the ridiculously low level of funds and personnel available to the UN made it virtually impossible to exert what little authority it had. By contrast, in Namibia, with a fifth of the population of Angola and a much less serious military problem, the UN spent 350 million dollars and deployed 7,000 people as part of the Transitional Arrangement Group (UNTAG). In Angola its budget was 130 million dollars and UNAVEM's staff numbers remained below 1,000 even at the height of its activity, when it provided 350 military observers, 90 police officers and 100 civilians, rising to 400 during the elections themselves. Without proper instruments to control its enforcement, the only guarantee of the peace process was the good faith of the parties themselves.

IMPLEMENTING THE AGREEMENTS: A WORK OF FICTION

The agreements were inherently unworkable and were in fact only partially or superficially implemented. Tension mounted as one violation followed another but the international community did not see fit to oversee the demobilization and disarming of the two warring sides: the UN contented itself with registering men and arms arriving at the demobilization camps and turned a blind eye to the hidden arms caches and soldiers outside the assembly areas. Thus the troika, seconded by the UN, acted as guarantors of an 'implementation' that was really a fiction in the face of the relentless pressure to hold elections at any price. Although UNITA kept its troops on a war footing, the MPLA created an 'anti-riot' police force and the unified army supposedly made up of soldiers from both sides remained at only a tenth of its planned strength, the troika and the UN solemnly pronounced the two armies to be disbanded and the unified army constituted. They then went on to organize the elections as though the sole objective of the peace process were to hold them on the planned date. As a result, the elections were held in an extremely polarized country with a government party hogging all the administrative resources and a militarized party panting to seize the reins of power. While none of the conditions necessary for the holding of free and fair elections had been met, all the ingredients for an explosion were in place: the fact that both sides had the means to contest the results with violence meant that the elections supposed to crown the peace process merely triggered off a new war.

The Namibian experience

A look at the implementation of Resolution 435 in Namibia between 1988 and 1990 offers a telling contrast to the Angolan operation in 1992. Namibia was a tricky operation for the UN, which had to juggle peacekeeping, assistance in decolonization and the transition to independence, and the withdrawal of Cuban troops from Angola.

The 7,000 soldiers, police officers and civilians making up the United Nations Transitional Arrangement Group (UNTAG) had a tough job: they had only the months between 1 April 1989, the start of the ceasefire between the South African army and PLAN, the armed wing of the liberation movement SWAPO, and 7 November, the date set for the election of Namibia's constituent assembly, to dampen down hostility between the two belligerents.

From the outset UNTAG proved powerless to halt disproportionate South African reprisals, notably one following a PLAN incursion into Namibia. This part of its mandate, plus demobilization and the withdrawal of South African police and military, was the hardest to implement, especially as the UN was unable to do anything about the continuing existence of militia not covered by Resolution 435. But UNTAG did manage to mount an effective guard over the reception camps for demobilized PLAN soldiers and the peace was kept. The return of 41,000 SWAPO exiles, the bulk of them by air in a total of 452 aircraft, did something to improve UNTAG's image in the minds of Namibians, who had hitherto felt that UNTAG was too eager to cooperate with South Africa. The combination of the massive deployment of observers and good logistics ensured the elections went smoothly. As a result, UNTAG's verdict on the elections, the only thing on which it really had any final say, had far greater weight than would that of the UN Angola Verification Mission (UNAVEM) two years later.

But we should not lose sight of the essential fact that South Africa, having successfully blocked application of Resolution 435 for ten years, remained in control of events right up to independence and obtained the departure of Cuban troops from Angola. At least the UN was successful in showing South Africa that force was not the only way to maintain a tight grip on the region – a strategy that may well have prompted moves to reach a settlement in South Africa itself.

THE SPIRAL OF VIOLENCE

The elections were held and all observers remarked on the enthusiasm and civic spirit displayed by Angolans, who turned out to express not just their fears but also their hopes for a lasting peace and the rule of law rather than force. But no sooner was its defeat clear than UNITA made accusations of 'massive and widespread fraud', put its war machine back on battle footing and demanded the annulment of the elections. In the face of UNITA's threats the UN proved powerless to enforce compliance with the election results and it was forced to watch helplessly as the MPLA launched a 'clean-up' operation in Luanda and other towns over the first weekend of November 1992. In the space of three days, massacres left thousands of people dead and irremediably returned the country to war.

This purge and the retaliatory massacres that followed marked the first large-scale involvement of civilians in the war, both as protagonists and victims, and a stepping-up of the ethnic polarization of the conflict. The desire for peace, shared by a majority of Angolans when the peace agreements were signed and manifest during the elections, gave way to despair and terror as political hatreds and ethnic fears gained the upper hand.

Hopes of a political solution have faded as the fighting intensifies and all attempts to get negotiations going have failed so far. While the international community is now ready to consider stepping up its presence in Angola, if only to salvage its image and credibility for other operations, it comes rather late for Angola. Above all, it comes late for the Angolan people, who are in the throes of a war that has become more destructive, more violent and more cruel than anything they have known before. In the space of a year, this fresh orgy of fighting has claimed tens of thousands of lives and tens of thousands have died of hunger, disease or sheer exhaustion as they struggled to reach a place of safety. Some two million people, about a fifth of the population, have been forced to flee their homes and are living in appalling conditions without proper food or sanitation. Life in the war zones is reduced to a struggle for survival. Virtually the whole country has become a war zone and only the capital and a few coastal areas have escaped. Towns that were places of refuge, however precarious, during the 'last' war are now in the thick of the fighting. Some have been under siege for months, cut off from the outside world, bombarded from the air and the ground, and short of water, medicines and food. It is impossible to farm because of mines and the danger of attack, and the sporadic deliveries of aid cover only part of their needs. Aid is not only held up by the fighting but is also a victim of politics. Both the government and UNITA want aid for 'their' people but are reluctant to allow aid to reach the other side for fear that it will end up in the hands of the opposing army. Requests made by relief organizations for flight authorizations go unanswered, the humanitarian aid corridors are not in place because the two sides will not guarantee the safety of convoys, and even the agreements that have been reached are often violated – planes carrying aid have been shot down by UNITA. Relief organizations too are now hostages to the warring parties.

INTERNATIONAL RESPONSIBILITY

The international community bears a terrible responsibility for the breakdown of the peace process it engineered and supervised at every step of the way. Its influence was decisive in the conduct of the negotiations and the content of the agreements and their implementation. The greatest responsibility must be borne by the troika countries, and especially the United States, which as mediators failed to demonstrate the necessary impartiality and pushed for unrealistic measures that carried the risk of war. The international community intervened in the name of democracy, but the democracy on offer was reduced to the holding of elections, which were seen merely as the last battle of the Angolan war. In flagrant violation of the agreements of which it was the guarantor, the international community did not even equip itself with a bare minimum of means to carry out its central task in pursuit of peace, namely the demilitarization and disarming of the belligerents.

The UN bears a share of the responsibility for the role it agreed to play in the process and for giving its stamp of approval to each stage on the way, thereby displaying its impotence and earning only discredit. Perhaps the lessons of this débâcle will be drawn in Mozambique since the Mozambican agreements are closely modelled on the Angolan ones. But in Angola the inherent weaknesses of the peace process and the failure of the international community to correct them have led the country down a blind alley. At best this peace operation has cost Angola the tragedy of a new war and inflicted wounds that will be difficult to heal. At worst, the international community will feel obliged either to withdraw from the Angolan 'mess' or to intervene on a massive scale that will surely make the political problem harder than ever to resolve.

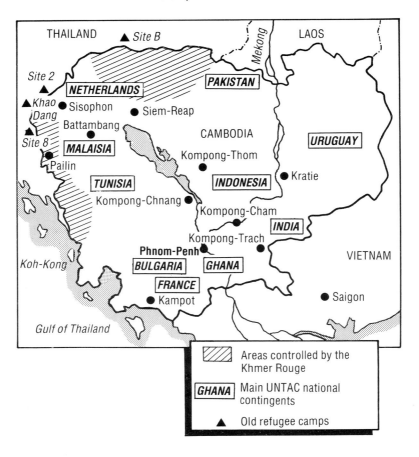

THAILAND ▲ Site B · Mekong · LAOS

Site 2 ▲ · PAKISTAN

NETHERLANDS

▲Khao ● Sisophon · ● Siem-Reap
¡Dang
▲ · Battambang ● · CAMBODIA · URUGUAY
Site 8
MALAISIA · Kompong-Thom ●

●Pailin · ● Kratie
INDONESIA
TUNISIA
Kompong-Chnang ● · INDIA
· Kompong-Cham ●

Kompong-Trach ●
Phnom-Penh● · VIETNAM
Koh-Kong · BULGARIA · GHANA

FRANCE · ● Saigon
● Kampot

Gulf of Thailand

▨ Areas controlled by the
Khmer Rouge

GHANA Main UNTAC national
contingents

▲ Old refugee camps

8

CAMBODIA
Elections in the killing fields

After two years of difficult negotiations, culminating in the signing of the Paris Agreements of 23 October 1991, more than twenty years of fighting came to an end in Cambodia with the implementation of one of the largest operations ever mounted by the United Nations. The high hopes raised by the Paris Agreements and the extraordinary commitment on the part of the international community was commensurate with the extent of the tragedy suffered by the people of Cambodia. However, a peace agreement, even one that is initialled by all five permanent members of the UN Security Council and thirteen other nations, is not the same thing as peace: two years on from the Paris Conference, men and women are still dying on the banks of the Mekong, and human rights violations continue unchecked. Democracy and the rule of law have undoubtedly gained ground, and the Cambodian people roundly rejected the ways of violence at the elections of 23–8 May 1983, but the danger of further bouts of bloody conflict, and indeed full-scale civil war, cannot yet be discounted. Despite being present in large numbers, UN personnel on the ground have failed to persuade the various factions to lay down their arms, nor has any solution been found to the Khmer Rouge problem.

CAMBODIA'S THREE WARS

In fact, over the last quarter of a century, Cambodia has had not one but three wars. The first began in the early 1960s, when communist guerrillas supported peasant farmers in their struggle against the regime of Norodom Sihanouk. In June 1970, three months after the overthrow of Sihanouk and his replacement by General Lon Nol, events took a spectacular turn for the worse when the United States, bogged down in Vietnam, decided to extend the war to Cambodia and launched a massive bombing campaign that claimed tens of thousands of victims and destroyed much of the country's infra-structure. This first war ended on 17 April 1975, with the victorious Khmer Rouge marching into Phnom Penh. The second started a few hours later, when the new masters of Cambodia ordered the immediate evacuation of the entire urban population. This exodus was the beginning of a Khmer Rouge campaign to exterminate all opposition, starting with the intellectuals, city-dwellers and all those who had been 'perverted' by contact with foreign cultures, moving on to anyone to whom the invisible and all-powerful Angkar, 'the organization', took a dislike. This genocide, which led to nearly a million deaths, came to an end on 7 January 1979 when, after months of border skirmishes, the Vietnamese army took Phnom Penh from the Khmer Rouge and replaced their 'Democratic Kampuchea' with a 'People's Republic of Kampuchea', under the aegis of the Hanoi regime. The third war was sparked by the exodus of hundreds of thousands of Cambodians fleeing from the fighting towards the Thai border, where the first refugee camps were hastily set up. This war, which was to last for more than ten years, pitted the Phnom Penh army and its Vietnamese protectors against a coalition backed by China, ASEAN, the United States and a number of European countries, and consisting of three political and military organizations: the Khmer Rouge, the Khmer People's National Liberation Front (KPNLF), under former Prime Minister Son Sann, and Sihanouk's United National Front for an Independent, Neutral, Peaceful and Cooperative Cambodia (FUNCINPEC).

UN: FROM INDIFFERENCE TO INTERVENTION

Having started in an era dominated by East–West conflict, against a backdrop of Sino-Vietnamese rivalry, at a time when South-East Asia was dividing into two hostile blocs, ASEAN and the three countries of Indo-China (Vietnam, Laos and Cambodia), the war in Cambodia was at first greeted with profound indifference by the United Nations. It was not until January 1979, and Vietnam's overthrow of the Pol Pot regime, that the UN, hitherto unmoved by the tragedy visited on the country by the Khmer Rouge, reacted to a perceived violation of the established international order, namely Vietnam's invasion of its neighbour. The Security Council at long last gave the issue some attention, adopting a series of resolutions urging the Secretary-General to follow up closely on the situation and propose his 'good offices' to promote a peaceful solution to the problem. However, in spite of their crimes, the Khmer Rouge continued to represent

What happened to reconstruction?

While the UN has spent nearly three billion dollars on its peace-keeping operation in Cambodia, rehabilitation and rebuilding programmes have had to make do with much less. Yet the needs of this devastated country are enormous: infrastructure is virtually non-existent, the road network is in a pitiful state, and the sanitary system is just about kept going through the efforts of nearly a hundred NGOs, the donor countries' preferred channel for aid pending the election of a recognized government.

The Tokyo conference of June 1992 raised great hopes: the donor countries approved the Secretary-General's recommend-ations and undertook to finance Cambodia's 'immediate needs' to the tune of 810 million dollars. One year on, disillusionment has set in: only a derisory proportion of the funds pledged has been disbursed – only 2.3 per cent of the financing promised for infrastructure, for example, and 13 per cent of the amount ear-marked for health projects. The opposition parties within the SNC have done their utmost to ensure that no payments are made to a government that the international community is wary of strengthening through financial aid.

UNTAC's 'rehabilitation department' never really got going, and was never able to carve out a niche for itself among the galaxy of UN agencies present in Cambodia, all competing for the same hand-outs. As for UNTAC's military forces, they were only deployed at a late stage in token, inexpensive 'civic action' operations.

The paradox of the most expensive operation ever mounted by the United Nations is that after two years it is leaving the country in exactly the same catastrophic condition as it found it in. For most of the population, the only economic consequence of the international presence in Cambodia will have been a significant rise in the cost of living and a spectacular increase in corruption and speculation. As the UN forces prepare to depart, the rebuilding of Cambodia has yet to get under way.

Cambodia at the United Nations for more than ten years. Only with the advent of perestroika, followed by the collapse of the Soviet Union, which deprived Vietnam of its mainstay and put an end to the Cold War, was the UN able to take the initiative and deploy its good offices with French and Indonesian backing. The withdrawal of Vietnamese troops began in 1986, and Prince Sihanouk and the Prime Minister engaged in talks in France, but it was to take a further five years of chaotic negotiation, under the auspices of the two co-sponsors of the peace process, France and Indonesia, to finalize the Paris Agreements. These texts laid down the full range of legal, military, administrative, political and diplomatic provisions that together made up a strategy for the transition to peace. The Supreme National Council (SNC), consisting of representatives of each of the four parties and presided over by Norodom Sihanouk, was defined as 'the unique legitimate body and source of authority in which, throughout the transitional period, the sovereignty, independence and unity of Cambodia are enshrined'. For a transitional period of twenty-one months power was vested in the United Nations Transitional Authority in Cambodia (UNTAC), with a budget of nearly three billion dollars. In November 1991, the deployment of more than 15,000 Blue Helmets, 3,600 police personnel and nearly 5,000 officials and civilians from 32 countries got under way. UNTAC's brief was five-fold: (1) to demobilize, disarm and canton 70 per cent of each party's military forces; (2) to create a 'neutral political environment' that would allow the 'free and fair' election of a constituent assembly; (3) to relaunch and rebuild Cambodia; (4) to repatriate and reintegrate the 350,000 refugees from the camps in Thailand; (5) to protect the sovereignty and integrity of Cambodia.

THE OBDURACY OF THE KHMER ROUGE

It would be putting it extremely mildly to say that these objectives have only been partially achieved. After more than fifteen years of international isolation the Cambodians had high hopes of the United Nations, but these were swiftly dashed by the tardy, poorly planned and badly coordinated arrival of contingents of widely differing calibre with little or no knowledge of Cambodian realities and often scant respect for local customs. Delays in deployment and the United Nations' inability to provide genuine administrative control soon sapped UNTAC's credibility. For a start, in spite of the commitments made when the Paris Agreements were signed, the Blue Helmets were unable to gain access to areas under Khmer Rouge control,

Human rights violations

Between November 1992 and March 1993, UNTAC's human rights department recorded more than a hundred serious human rights violations. This figure is clearly nowhere near accurate: large numbers of incidents go unreported, particularly where members of the Phnom Penh administration are implicated, and most violations in the areas under Khmer Rouge control are never recorded.

None of the four parties to the conflict leading up to the Paris Agreements (i.e., the Phnom Penh regime, FUNCINPEC, KPNLF and the Khmer Rouge) are above criticism when it comes to human rights violations. However, the chief culprits are the Khmer Rouge, who have never renounced their old ways in the areas under their control, and who are responsible for a series of racist attacks on Vietnamese villages that have resulted in large numbers of deaths. The Phnom Penh regime renounced Marxist-Leninism in 1991, but its institutions and methods have remained those of a totalitarian state.

The United Nations ultimately attached only minimal priority to the issue of human rights – witness the poor allocation of funds and human resources to the relevant department. To its credit, UNTAC managed to persuade the SNC to ratify a number of treaties, secured the release of hundreds of political prisoners, supported the first independent Cambodian human rights movements and launched a major educational programme in this field. However, it proved incapable of conducting enquiries into violations and apprehending their perpetrators, even when their identity was known. Abuses continued unchecked and unpunished through- out the transitional period, so anxious was UNTAC to avoid giving offence to any of the factions in its concern to keep the peace process on the rails. Gravely underestimating the legacy of violence and anarchy, the United Nations never really tried to lay the foundations for establishing the rule of law.

accounting for around 15 per cent of the country. On the pretext that Vietnamese units remained in Cambodia, Khmer Rouge leaders refused to disarm and canton their forces under UN supervision. The

UN's sole reaction to this flagrant violation of the Paris Agreements was to issue a series of increasingly weak ultimatums that stripped it of all credibility and exposed the Blue Helmets to mounting pressure and humiliation. As a result of Khmer Rouge obduracy, the disarmament of the other three factions, and particularly the Phnom Penh army, was also suspended.

The main consequence of the Blue Helmets' military and political impotence, which allowed the factions to keep most of their arms, was the *de facto* division of Cambodia into two parts: one, under UNTAC control, where, in spite of incidents causing a considerable number of deaths, it was possible to organize voter registration and the elections themselves in a more or less orderly fashion, and the other, under the control of the Khmer Rouge, where the people were denied any chance of expressing themselves. UNTAC's meek acquiescence also allowed the Khmer Rouge, with the active complicity of Thailand, to continue their looting of the country's natural resources, particularly timber and rubies, while the other three parties followed their example through Laos and Vietnam. In other words, UNTAC failed miserably to 'protect Cambodia's integrity', as it failed to 'create a neutral political environment' in the face of Khmer Rouge obduracy and the bad faith of the Phnom Penh regime. The administrative apparatus of the Cambodian state, which in the absence of effective UN supervision retained its power, was transformed into an electoral propaganda machine and engine of intimidation acting on behalf of Prime Minister Hun Sen's Cambodian People's Party. On the other hand, in spite of some poor planning, the repatriation of refugees has proved to be one of the UN's rare success stories, thanks to the personal commitment of the local UNHCR representative. Nevertheless, attempts to promote the reintegration of returnees have had to contend with major obstacles, primarily linked to the serious dearth of mine-clearing facilities and the continuing atmosphere of insecurity in rural areas. As in many other countries, the UN in Cambodia has failed to rid the country of mines, which not only prolong the ravages of war well into the peace process, but also represent one of the main obstacles to peace itself.

CAMBODIA AND ITS DEMONS

In the absence of any real determination on the part of UNTAC and without adequate support from the main donor countries, the 'relaunching' of the country, which was supposed to be the first phase of rebuilding, has hardly got off the ground. The international community's contribution to economic renewal has basically remained confined to the rain of dollars showered on Cambodia by the 22,000 members of UNTAC. This temporary drip-feed has succeeded only in generating corruption, speculation and inflation: the exchange rate of the riel against the dollar collapsed within a year, while the cost of fish and meat has risen five-fold, further exacerbating the inequality between town and country. The main beneficiaries of this largesse have been Thai and Chinese traders: apart from a handful of corrupt speculators, politicians and officials, the local economy has received only a very modest slice of the cake, while the Cambodian people have had to cope with the shock of a multinational invasion that, although peaceful, has not always respected their traditions and culture as it should. One of UNTAC's main tasks was to guarantee respect for human rights in Cambodia, but it has been unable to rid the country of the prevailing anarchy and the blight of political violence. A number of human rights organizations have sprung up over the past two years, but the UN has proved incapable of setting up an embryonic independent legal system or of countering the Khmer Rouge's racist propaganda and the slaughter of Vietnamese civilians. Furthermore, the UN troops themselves do not have impeccable human rights credentials either, and accusations of brutality and rape by some UN soldiers have been punished only with light disciplinary measures by the commanders of the contingents concerned. The multinational character of the UN military and police forces, a consequence of the 'national quotas' principle, has been particularly burdensome in Cambodia, where a number of undisciplined and poorly trained contingents have flatly refused to carry out their appointed tasks. The fact that the police force is made up of officers from democratic countries – accustomed to observing legal procedure and human rights – working alongside officers supplied by authoritarian regimes, has been another negative factor, often aggravated by communication problems: in February 1993, the UN's 3,600 police officers between them spoke a total of twenty different languages!

In Cambodia the UN has behaved as if its sole objective was to organize elections at the appointed time; as if the restoration of territorial integrity and national sovereignty, the reconstruction of the country, the establishment of the rule of law and the demobilization and disarmament of the factions could be taken care of at a later date. The elections were indeed held at the appointed time and, against all expectations, without violence, with Sihanouk gaining a slender majority over the party in power. This unexpected success is the UN's crowning achievement, but the atmosphere of uncertainty persists, against a backdrop of fighting in the provinces, insecurity, human rights violations and the ongoing pillage of Cambodia's resources by its neighbours. Enabling the Cambodian people, who have never enjoyed the political rights that are taken for granted in democratic countries, to choose their own representatives was undoubtedly one of UNTAC's main tasks, but it was not the only one. In the absence of a clearly-defined strategy and without the firm backing of the international community, the UN was a prisoner of both its ponderous bureaucracy and its 'diplomacy of patience'. Somewhere along the line it forgot its mandate, and only achieved a very small part of the task it was appointed to carry out in Cambodia under the Paris Agreements. By bringing its presence on the ground to an end, having secured neither the disarmament of the Khmer Rouge nor genuine political stability, the UN is leaving Cambodia prey to its old demons.

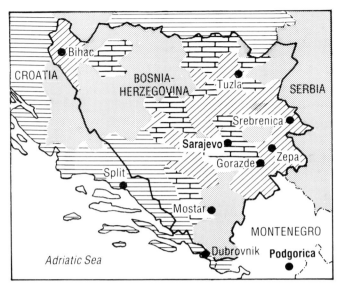

Bosnia before the war (1981 census); areas comprising:

Over 50 per cent Serb	Over 50 per cent Croat
Over 50 per cent Moslem	Mixed

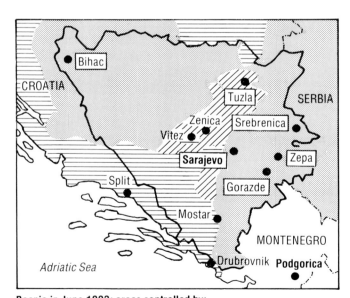

Bosnia in June 1993; areas controlled by:

Serbs	Croats
Moslems	Gorazde Towns declared 'UN security zones'

9

BOSNIA
The soft option

The policy adopted by the Western powers in April 1992, at the outbreak of the war in Bosnia-Herzegovina, was tantamount to accepting the disappearance of a state they had just recognized. Without reflection or prior public debate, they decided not to use force, choosing instead to treat the situation in Bosnia as a humanitarian crisis. The Security Council became a forum in which the West's leaders drew up a series of unconvincing measures aimed at helping the victims and punishing the aggressors. Eighteen months later, the disastrous results of this policy are plain to see. By hesitating, the international community has left the aggressors a clear field, content to follow in their wake with relief convoys that get through only when the attackers see fit. More than 200,000 Bosnians have died, most of them Muslims, and 2,300,000 people have been forced out of their homes by a policy of terror pursued with impunity in the face of an impotent international community.

CROATIA: PEACEKEEPING MAINTAINS THE *STATUS QUO*

The international community's failure is essentially a consequence of the inability of Europe and the United States to agree on a common definition of the post-Cold War world order. Worried by the dismemberment of the Soviet Union and hoping to prevent Yugoslavia from breaking up, the West's major powers set their faces against outside intervention when the Yugoslav army reacted to declarations of independence from Croatia and Slovenia by bombarding Croatia. This stance was interpreted in Belgrade as a green light for the use of force; by the end of 1991, Serb militias, backed by the Belgrade-controlled Yugoslav National Army, had conquered a quarter of Croatia's territory. The January 1992 ceasefire negotiated by the UN special envoy, Cyrus Vance, marked the beginning of the UN's gradual involvement on the ground in former Yugoslavia, with the deployment in Croatia of a protection force (UNPROFOR) intended to enforce the 'Vance plan'. This 14,000 strong force was supposed to disband and disarm the militias, supervise the withdrawal of the Yugoslav National Army and help 500,000 displaced persons return to the protected areas. In addition, 600 UN policemen were given the task of safeguarding human rights, with a theoretical mandate to register complaints and investigate offences. However, the drawbacks of this conventional peacekeeping force soon became apparent: though intended as an interim authority, pending a political solution, it had no effective means of fulfilling its mandate, since there was no clear political direction from the West. Though effectively preventing the renewal of fighting between Serbs and Croats in the Krajina, UNPROFOR's presence actually maintained the *status quo*, freezing the military situation to the advantage of the Serb militias, which proceeded to set up a government. Moreover, the slow deployment of the UN peacekeepers permitted the Serb militias to complete their 'ethnic cleansing': once in place, although the United Nations were pleased to report the end of the 'clean-up', in fact all non-Serbs had by then been killed or driven out, and the new police force was simply the old militia in new uniforms. Disarmament and demobilization were soon forgotten, and not one of the 500,000 refugees was able to return home. The safety of the UN contingents very soon became more important than protecting civilians, and the deployment of UNPROFOR troops seemed to become an end in itself.

THE BOSNIAN QUAGMIRE

The implications of the deployment of UN forces in Croatia did not go unnoticed: the deterrent value of UN troops, though present in Bosnia before the fighting started, was annulled by their loss of credibility in Croatia and the Western countries' lack of political resolve. Throughout the tragedy, those responsible for the war would capitalize on the western community's vacillation and internal divisions. The offensive launched against the new state by Serb nationalists on 6 April 1992, in the hope of building a Greater Serbia on the ruins of the old multinational Yugoslavia, just pre-empted Bosnia's international recognition in May. But recognition is not support, and the Western powers rejected the Bosnian government's appeals for assistance, dismissed the possibility of military intervention and enforced an arms embargo that penalized only the Bosnians, since their assailants were already well equipped. Although largely made up of Bosnian

Plenty of resolutions, no resolve

Although the UN Security Council has adopted thirty or so resolutions in regard to former Yugoslavia, this whole period will go down in history as one of the UN's most shameful periods of self-imposed impotence. The gulf between words and action was highlighted as never before: the UN's highest decision-making authority has acted as though the adoption of a resolution were an end in itself, regardless of whether or not it is ever implemented.

In any other situation the exercise would be laughable. Here, the solemn recording of hollow consensus only underlines the members' lack of political resolve. How else can one account for the need for at least three resolutions before enforcing an embargo, a no-fly zone or a protected area?

Resolution 781 will remain a text-book case. Adopted on 9 October 1992, it bans flights over Bosnia-Herzegovina. Six months and 500 violations of Bosnian airspace later, the Security Council at last decided to act on its initial decision. Resolution 816 finally authorized the dispatch of NATO aircraft to enforce the no-fly zone.

At least this was a second resolution that backed up the first. Resolution 770, adopted by the Security Council on 13 August 1992, was not so lucky. And yet it concerned the Serb detention camps, which had so shocked the world, and referred to the use of 'all necessary measures' to have them closed. Several months later, these camps were still in place, prompting France, in early 1993, to threaten to liberate them alone, although this, too, came to nothing.

Resolution 836 of 4 June 1993, establishing protected areas under international protection in the last Muslim pockets, was no more successful. Week after week, the inhabitants of these areas waited in vain for the peacekeeping forces supposed to protect them. Had they not been warned that the Security Council's resolutions were anything but resolute?

Serbs, the attacking forces were, in fact, equipped, trained and supported by the predominantly Serb army of what remained of Yugoslavia under the leadership of Slobodan Milosevic. The international community's initiatives have been a catalogue of inertia and indecision, serving only to highlight the gulf between words and action. Examples include the economic sanctions voted against the new Yugoslavia on 27 April 1992 and first applied eleven months later, or the ban on flights over Bosnian airspace adopted by the Security Council on 9 October 1992 and first enforced on 31 March 1993, six months later.

Meanwhile, in Bosnia, the strategy of 'ethnic cleansing' of Muslims and Croats was pursued through a succession of massacres and atrocities: the shelling of civilians, the manipulation of food supplies to create organized starvation, the selective destruction of villages and districts, arbitrary arrest, torture, systematic rape, summary execution and the forced transfer of hundreds of thousands of people were the chief instruments of a policy of terror aimed at driving people from their homes and controlling conquered territories by methods sometimes reminiscent of the Third Reich. Yet Western leaders did not speak out until August 1992, when public outcry at reports of concentration camps forced them to react before playing down the scale of the allegations. The gravity of the presumed atrocities was, however, acknowledged nine months later by the Security Council, with the adoption, on 25 May 1993, of Resolution 827, which set up the first international war crimes tribunal since Nuremberg. But nothing has been done to put an end to the crimes, and the lack of human and material resources for the new tribunal suggests that the measure was largely cosmetic.

THE DIPLOMACY OF IMPOTENCE

The joint EC–UN initiative led by Cyrus Vance and Lord Owen further illustrates the West's spinelessness in the face of military aggression. In August and September 1992, the two mediators drew up a complex peace plan, which, though providing for the partition of Bosnia into ten provinces and robbing the central government of almost all authority, did obstruct the Serbs in their principal war aim, namely the establishment of a corridor between Serbia and Serb enclaves in Croatia and Bosnia. The first to accept was the tiny self-proclaimed Bosnian Croat state of 'Herceg-Bosna', headed by Mate Boban, a protégé of the Croatian leader, Franjo Tudjman; it was followed by the mainly Muslim government of Aliya Izetbegovic. But the Bosnian

The Srebrenica fraud

The suffering endured by the people of Srebrenica, a Muslim enclave in Bosnia, besieged and bombarded for over a year, illustrates the limitations and ambiguities of UN 'humanitarian' operations in former Yugoslavia.

While Resolution 770 provided for all necessary measures to assist the delivery of humanitarian assistance, access to the victims continued to depend on the say-so of the factions. The passage of aid convoys remained subject to prior authorization from the Serbs controlling the territory and the local commanders holding the bridge at Zvornik, the gateway to Srebrenica. In early 1993, UNPROFOR was held at bay for weeks, while the situation deteriorated in the overcrowded enclave: there was a shortage of food for the town's 9,000 inhabitants and the 30,000 Muslims who had sought refuge there.

When the humanitarian organizations did finally get into Srebrenica in late March 1993, they found themselves facing a terrible dilemma. No sooner were the lorries unloaded than they were swamped by people desperate to flee. Should they help civilians by evacuating them, at the risk of contributing to 'ethnic cleansing'? Faced with the distress of the population, the UNHCR decided to evacuate people, under the sardonic gaze of the Serbs, who could not have hoped for more.

When, in April 1993, Srebrenica was declared a 'protected area', it discovered the gulf between the adoption and application of a Security Council resolution. Although Resolutions 819, 824 and 836 'resolved' to promote the withdrawal of all military units but those of the government of the Republic of Bosnia-Herzegovina, the peacekeepers were denied access to the enclave until they had signed an agreement with the Serbs for the unilateral disarmament of the Muslims. The besieging forces gradually strangled the town, allowing only a trickle of humanitarian aid through and refusing anything that might help improve the longer-term living conditions in a town that has become a prison.

Serbs, under the leadership of Radovan Karadzic, scuppered the plan. A third of Bosnia's population, they had seized control of over 70 per cent of its territory and saw no reason to settle for the 43 per cent offered by the two negotiators. The abandonment of this patchwork in the summer of 1993 in favour of the old plan based on the cantonization of Bosnia on ethnic lines saw the conflict come full circle. Setback followed setback, with one day's unaccept- able solutions becoming the next day's proposals: this diplomatic 'solution' formally acknowledged the carve-up of Bosnia along ethnic lines, reducing it to a figurehead and paving the way for the dis- mantling of the country by the annexation, open or covert, of the Serb and Croat cantons to their neighbouring mother countries. And what would become of the Muslims, refugees in their own land?

THE HUMANITARIAN ILLUSION

Unable to deter the aggressor, powerless to defend a recognized state or press for a political settlement, the international community has been equally unable to fulfil its self-conferred humanitarian mandate. Even in this limited domain, its initiatives have all too often been impulsive or media-driven, a failing only concealed from the public by UNHCR's spectacular airbridge to Sarajevo. Instructed by the United Nations to handle humanitarian aid in Bosnia, UNHCR has fulfilled its task to the best of its ability, limited by the combined effects of the determination of the warring parties and the feebleness of the major powers. The deployment of UN peacekeeping troops to protect aid convoys (UNPROFOR 2) was strikingly slow: four months after the war began, there were still only 1,700 men in the field. On 13 August 1992 the Security Council voted to send a further 6,000 troops to protect aid convoys, but they did not arrive until the end of October and were not mandated to protect civilians. As if the myriad diffi- culties of the field operation and the negotiations were not enough, the UN operation has been constantly obstructed by conflicts between member states and disputes between the Secretariat-General and field officials about the scope of the mandate. Security Council Resolution 770 authorizes the peacekeepers to take all necessary measures to ensure the delivery of humanitarian aid, but the UN has throughout the crisis imposed a narrow interpretation of the mandate: when faced with the choice of using force or negotiation to gain access to victims, it has opted for the latter, the lack of political resolve and resources leaving it little choice in the matter. The peacekeepers have consequently found themselves subject to the whims of the militias, becoming hostages to the warring parties. The UN forces, dispatched to protect humanitarian aid deliveries, have been shackled by a restrictive interpretation of their mandate that prevents them defending aid organizations – and sometimes even themselves. Considering that troops are present, the conditions in which relief workers are operating in the field has been a grotesque parody of what is tolerable, even in a war. Convoys from humanitarian organizations passing through checkpoints to bring aid to people in desperate need have often been harassed, threatened or pillaged by the militias, sometimes before the very eyes of UNPROFOR soldiers, watching passively from their armoured vehicles. The UN has been unable to set up regular road convoys to besieged towns or threatened areas, which have to make do with air drops of food by American planes. Appointed by the international community to coordinate relief operations in former Yugoslavia, UNHCR has attempted to defend certain fundamental principles. But when it decided, in February 1993, to suspend its operations to show that it would not stand for the obstruction of humanitarian operations, it was disowned by the Secretary-General, and access to the victims became more problematic than ever. Restricted to supply operations, the volume and frequency of which are dictated by the aggressors, such 'humanitarian diplomacy' has reduced aid to a tactical bargaining chip, and diplomacy to a parody of dialogue, in which principles are sacrificed for transient benefits and sterile agreements.

By spring 1993, the Bosnian State was no more than a series of isolated enclaves, such as Sarajevo, Gorazde and Srebrenica, and the only question was whether they would survive. The Bosnian Croats, who controlled the land routes to the outside world, broke their alliance with the Muslims and began to block all convoys, with the aim of seizing the territory allotted to them by the Vance–Owen plan. The Muslims counter-attacked, making the war even more complex than before. Confronted with this situation, the United States, the United Kingdom, France and the other powers adopted a proposal to set up UN-protected areas in a dozen towns and regions surrounded by Serb forces, but failed once again to equip themselves with the wherewithal to implement these decisions.

The case of Srebrenica is most revealing: it took months and the determination of General Morillon for the UN to gain access to the besieged town. With the Serbs refusing to stop bombarding the 50,000 civilians until all had been disarmed, the Canadian UN forces unilaterally disarmed the town's defenders. Despite the presence of 150 Canadian soldiers, Srebrenica has remained under siege, held in a stranglehold by the Serbs and utterly dependent on their say-so for supplies and safety. The evacuation of several thousand people, most of them refugees from other enclaves in eastern Bosnia, was regarded by the Bosnian authorities as a less harsh form of 'ethnic cleansing'. The UNPROFOR troops are in fact no more than observers: they 'observe' that there are wounded, that the Serbs have blown up the water-treatment plant outside town, that the winter is going to be harsh, but are unable to do anything more. Inside the besieged town, living conditions remain extremely difficult: fifteen to twenty people share five square metres and everyone survives on international aid. Cement and fuel, declared 'war materials' by the Serbs, are not allowed into the town, banishing any thought of rebuilding. The message from the besieging army to the inhabitants is clear: the protected areas were an illusion, their inhabitants have simply obtained a stay of execution, kept alive in their prison by the humanitarian organizations.

ALL PRINCIPLES RENOUNCED

As so often before in this riven country, the power of diplomacy has been harnessed to public relations, providing a backdrop for pious declarations, while the real drama takes place in the wings. Pending measures to 'save' Srebrenica, Sarajevo, Tuzla, Gorazde and the other enclaves, the cost of all those lost opportunities is increasing all the time. In the absence of a just settlement, the war in Bosnia-Herzegovina threatens to drag on for years in one form or another, with the risk that it might spread well beyond Yugoslavia. The establishment of camps for 'displaced persons', driven by terror from their homes under the eyes of a Europe more willing to appease than to enforce what is right, bodes ill for the future. Moreover, not only have most European countries caved in in the face of a policy of terror and systematic violation of the most basic human rights, they also try to deter the victims of the conflict from seeking refuge in the West. The Bosnian disaster has not only done serious damage to the credibility of the United Nations and its law-enforcement and security instruments, it has also seriously eroded the principles of the Geneva Conventions, as well as human rights values and the UN Convention on Genocide. In short, it has flouted all the ideals on which the European democracies were founded in the aftermath of the Second World War. Until some decision is taken, the citizens of prosperous Europe will have to look on, in anguish, as armed men continue to turn this small part of European civilization into a graveyard.

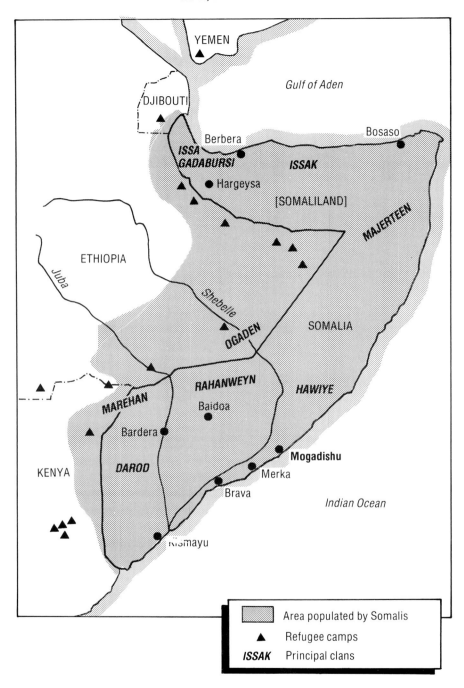

YEMEN

Gulf of Aden

DJIBOUTI

Berbera

Bosaso

ISSA GADABURSI

ISSAK

Hargeysa

[SOMALILAND]

MAJERTEEN

ETHIOPIA

Juba

Shebelle

OGADEN

SOMALIA

RAHANWEYN

HAWIYE

MAREHAN

Baidoa

Bardera

Mogadishu

Merka

DAROD

KENYA

Brava

Indian Ocean

Kismayu

	Area populated by Somalis
▲	Refugee camps
ISSAK	Principal clans

10

SOMALIA
Humanitarian aid outgunned

Somalia has been in the grip of an unprecedented crisis for the last three years. During this time, we have seen the disintegration of the country, the collapse of government and the breakdown of society. After twenty years of bloody dictatorship, a bitter war broke out in January 1991, causing a terrible famine. It was months before the international community decided to react, but indifference soon gave way to intervention. Following the failure of an initial contingent of Blue Helmets in autumn 1992, a large expeditionary force landed in Mogadishu in December. Five months later the United Nations took over only to be sucked into a military stand-off which now threatens to stifle the humanitarian concerns which were the reason for international intervention in the first place.

UNPRECEDENTED CHAOS

On 27 January 1991 Siad Barre fled Mogadishu after his final defeat in a vicious war, leaving behind a capital in ruins and a country bled dry. The dictator's fall was not enough to restore peace, however: the uprising against Siad Barre's regime soon gave way to fighting between factions which sent the country hurtling into a spiral of violence and destruction. From November 1991 to March 1992 the 'war of Mogadishu' dealt the capital a final blow, reducing it to a heap of rubble where looting and indiscriminate shooting were the rule. Throughout the entire country people fled the fighting or sought refuge in neighbouring countries in an attempt to find a means for survival and some degree of safety. Over 500,000 refugees arrived in Kenya, Ethiopia and even Yemen. In the south, hundreds of thousands of displaced people desperately tried to escape the constant harassment of pick-up trucks bristling with machine guns. The incessant fighting and slaughter, the systematic looting and destruction, and the constant to-ing and fro-ing of terrorized people gradually turned scarcity into shortages and shortages into famine. Disaster finally struck in early 1992 and within a few months hundreds of thousands of people were to die of hunger in a country abandoned to its fate and the rule of force.

UNITED NATIONS PARALYSED

In the first few months of the crisis, the international community was conspicuous by its absence: the fighting which preceded Siad Barre's fall resulted in the evacuation of the embassies and United Nations offices and, for almost a year and a half, a handful of humanitarian organizations were the only source of help. Until spring 1992, when a permanent representative of the Secretary-General arrived in Mogadishu, the UN agencies confined their efforts to minor evaluation sorties from their Nairobi offices. It was not until June that UNICEF set up a permanent team in Mogadishu. Faced with chronic insecurity and chaos, the UN had great difficulty in becoming operational: while the food aid required in spring 1992 was assessed at over 50,000 tonnes a month, the ICRC was left to assume virtually the sole responsibility for food distribution until the autumn, despite the fact that it was clearly unable to meet such massive requirements.

The United Nations agencies, more used to dealing with national governments, had great difficulty adapting to the lack of official representatives and were paralysed by coordination problems: the UNDP, a mainstay of the UN system, asserted its automatic right to take charge of coordination; UNICEF, the first agency in the field, claimed precedence while the DHA, recently set up to coordinate in emergencies, tried in vain to impose itself. In the end everyone decided to be their own coordinator with the result that the agencies each launched uncoordinated, and in most cases unsuitable, assistance programmes. Consequently, private humanitarian aid organizations still had to offset these shortcomings by carrying on with assistance programmes out of all proportion to their means while in July 1992 the United States arranged an emergency airlift from Kenya to do something about the unprecedented famine which had been devastating the country for six months. An initial aid plan drawn up by the United Nations in summer 1992 had hardly any impact and a new 100-day plan launched in October did not do much better.

Following the ceasefire agreed in March 1992 by the warlords of Mogadishu, the UN Security Council decided on 24 April to deploy 50 observers and a security force of 500 Blue Helmets as part of

The traps of military protection of relief aid

Under Resolution 794 the main objective of the international contingent is 'to establish a secure environment for humanitarian relief operations in Somalia'.

Since Siad Barre fell, the climate of insecurity has been the main obstacle to humanitarian aid in Somalia: it prevents the people trapped by the fighting from being reached and places aid organizations at the mercy of the looters. The humanitarian organizations which arrived in Somalia in 1991 had to recruit armed guards not only for their protection but simply to function. Although it meant going against their principles and promoting the war economy, they decided to pay a force to ward off attacks in an attempt to bring relief to the people most under threat.

The international operation upset this precarious balance of negotiated safety and replaced it by oppressive military protection. The humanitarian organizations were the first to be affected by partial and ineffective measures to disarm the armed bands which continued their activities in the very centre of Mogadishu and stepped up their ambushes on the country's roads. As a result of this greater vulnerability, since the supplies they were handling made the aid agencies the main target of banditry, a number of members of humanitarian organizations have died.

The increased insecurity has made the humanitarian organizations increasingly dependent on the protection afforded by the foreign forces without allowing them to forgo Somali armed protection and break the cycle of racketeering that goes with it. The need to act in conjunction with the military has created a situation where it is difficult to act independently and impartially. The confusion between military and humanitarian is ever greater in the minds of the Somalis and could prove disastrous. Now that the UN forces have joined the fighting in Somalia, the environment for humanitarian relief operations is more insecure than ever.

UNOSOM 1. Most of the observers did not arrive until July, however, and the Secretary-General's representative, Mohammed Sahnoun, who had had great difficulty negotiating the deployment of 500 Blue Helmets with the warlords, learnt from the BBC of the arrival of an additional 2,500 men. After a long absence, the UN had lost patience and seemed resolved to do without the warlords' agreement. The resignation-cum-dismissal of Mohammed Sahnoun in November 1992, following his public criticism of the UN agencies' inaction, put an abrupt end to the strategy of dialogue and negotiation skilfully conducted in the preceding months by the Secretary-General's representative. The situation then deteriorated rapidly: ships carrying relief aid were bombed or prevented from docking and attacks by looters became widespread. Lawlessness increased, with the warlords stepping up terrorist attacks against each other under the eyes of powerless Blue Helmets. Finally, the UN, which staked its last hopes on international intervention, risked an unverified claim, that 80 per cent of the aid was being hijacked. The massive public emotion aroused when the television cameras belatedly revealed the famine in July 1992 pushed the United States to send in troops.

THE US INTERVENTION

On 3 December 1992, UN Security Council Resolution 794 authorized the Secretary-General and the member states contributing to the international forces 'to use all necessary means to establish a secure environment for humanitarian relief operations in Somalia as soon as possible'. This Resolution gave the signal for the first major humanitarian policing operation since the end of the Cold War and authorized the use of force. Over 30,000 soldiers were to be mobilized in Operation Restore Hope under US command and on 9 December the first Marines landed in Mogadishu in the full glare of the world's television cameras.

The troops sent by the UN were not expected to have any difficulty in commanding the respect of the teenagers armed with kalashnikovs who were spreading terror in Somalia. This optimism, born of complete ignorance of the gravity and the nature of the crisis in Somalia, was quickly dispelled by the first violent incidents and disagreement on how the mandate should be interpreted.

While the UN insisted that disarming the combatants was essential for security, the US command defined the mission strictly in humanitarian terms. The US interpretation, which left aside the crucial problem of a political settlement, fitted in well with its ambitious

The impunity of the use of force

On 27 July 1993, UN Security Council Resolution 814 authorized the use of force in Somalia in order to restore peace, making the country a guinea pig for international action.

For the first time, the UN authorized its representatives to use force, not for dissuasion or self-defence, but for an offensive operation. However, the UN machinery for the use of force is incomplete and thus has never been used. Certain bodies provided for in the Charter, such as the Military Staff Committee, have never been set up. Their lack is now being felt. In Somalia the UN is not above the law – it is itself lawless.

The UN is used to acting as a buffer, but it has not equipped itself with an instrument to lay down limits for the use of force. It now stands accused of violating the laws of war and humanity. Sent in as liberators, the Blue Helmets have started to behave as yet another faction.

By attacking the humanitarian organizations' installations, blocking access to hospitals and crushing demonstrations by unarmed civilians, the UN is placing itself above the laws of war and claiming immunity in order to use what force it sees fit.

Orders are given by the UN and carried out by national contingents. In Somalia, the military is headless and the chain of responsibility has been broken. With no body to investigate, judge and punish its own abuses of power, the UN is displaying legal and operational irresponsibility.

An appeal sent by NGOs to the UN and the commanders of the national forces in Somalia, and a report by the US Department of Justice formally denounce this situation. These steps have been taken to impress on the UN that it is required to observe the laws of war and the rules set out in the Geneva Conventions for the use of force. The UN must also set up the bodies and create the system needed to ensure compliance with these laws, make them widely known and ensure that they are observed by the UN's own troops.

timetable to start withdrawing American troops as early as January and its commitment to 'zero casualties', an approach influenced by the lack of conviction behind a media-driven intervention.

In the beginning, military logistics outweighed any other con-sideration: the unloading of war equipment clogged up the port so that food consignments to the interior were held up even though some food-aid stocks were running out. After a few weeks, however, operations in the port were speeded up, mines were cleared from the main roads, food convoys were protected and food distribution stepped up. Since the famine had reached a peak in the summer of 1992 and the most vulnerable had already died, Restore Hope was not the only factor in helping to establish some degree of normality but, by removing most of the obstacles to the regular delivery of aid, it managed to speed it up.

While international intervention brought about a spectacular up-swing in relief operations, it did not achieve its security objective. Although things appeared more normal, there was still a great deal of insecurity and this was the main concern of the humanitarian organizations. The slowness of troop deployment and the lack of a coordinated policy on disarmament allowed the Somali private armies to hide with complete impunity. Moreover, the strategy of con-centrating troops for their own safety only created islands of security with armed bands and looters operating outside. While these islands were only relatively safe, looting was on the increase in Mogadishu and in many other towns even amidst a spectacular show of military equipment. Despite all their resources, the international forces did not succeed in making a large area safe for any length of time.

This poor result is largely accounted for by ignorance about Somali society, widely seen as a kind of wasteland swarming with armed thugs, a lack of understanding of the war economy and above all a tendency to focus on short-term solutions to the detriment of a real strategy for disarming the factions and the search for a political solution.

These failures were all the more worrying in that, apart from the ongoing violence and looting, the fighting was continuing, even in the regions theoretically under the control of international forces. In February 1993 General Morgan, Siad Barre's son-in-law, went into Kismayu and in a few weeks flushed out the partisans of Colonel Jess, who had just been disarmed by the international forces. This *coup*, accomplished under the very noses of the Belgian paratroopers and the US contingent deployed in the town, dealt a severe blow to the credibility of the international forces, which for the first time lost the semblance of neutrality. In turn, the position of the humanitarian organizations was made more precarious, as the Somalis came to associate them with the military force that, while supposedly humanitarian, was now seen as a party to the conflict.

THE RETURN OF THE UNITED NATIONS

In March 1993 the Security Council adopted Resolution 814, which called for the deployment of 28,000 Blue Helmets to take over from the UNITAF forces. The UN forces were thus given a broad mandate, particularly for disarming the warlords, under Chapter VII of the Charter: for the first time the UN was to get involved in an operation which could take it beyond peacekeeping – into peacemaking. And for the first time the United States committed troops under the UN flag, although it remained in charge of the operation, particularly with the appointment of Admiral Howe to overall command. The UNOSOM 2 mandate covered the whole of Somalia and embraced not only humanitarian aid but also the repatriation of refugees, resettlement of displaced persons, establishment of a police force, mine clearance, disarming the factions, the political reconciliation process, the reconstruction of the country and the rebuilding of its institutions.

The transition from international intervention under US command to a new UN operation, mooted since January and decided in March, did not actually take place until the beginning of May. The transition was a difficult one: the Blue Helmets had to take over Operation Restore Hope and regain the credibility lost by the UN over the previous two years. The UN's Somali record bore two major black marks: it had abandoned the country at the height of the fighting in 1991, then it had failed to take action when the famine was at its worst in 1992. Lastly, the first 500 Blue Helmets, far from protecting the supply of humanitarian aid, had themselves sought the protection of Somali armed guards. The United States was anxious to withdraw its troops but the deployment of new forces was the subject of lengthy negotiations further slowed down by the UN's cumbersome bureaucracy, problems of determining the chain of command and the crucial question of political support for such a peacemaking operation.

Once the famine was checked, the main aid objectives were to deal with the one and a half million displaced persons and refugees still completely dependent on foreign aid, to rebuild the infrastructure and secure economic recovery. The UN agencies, which were in the best position to work out a national reconstruction plan, were once again shackled by operational and recruitment problems. Despite the absence of government representatives and a fluid situation, they kept most of their staff in the Mogadishu offices and did not send enough experienced senior staff to the provinces. Up to May 1993, this bureaucratic approach was expressed in the launching of any number of unrelated emergency projects, before a proper strategy emerged, suited to the country's needs.

The absence of long-term policies is particularly worrying in the political sphere. It has been obvious since December 1992 that the international community's intervention lacked a political goal. Seen at first as a quick mopping-up operation, international intervention has assumed a longer-term perspective since March 1992, but the political objectives remain hazy and the national reconciliation process is making no headway. It is true that the crisis in Somalia was very complex, that the fabric of the country had collapsed and that it is questionable whether people from outside were qualified to suggest solutions in a country where government had never been more than a thin veneer imposed on society. Nevertheless, the international community's actions were rather puzzling: after legitimizing the clan leaders by giving them a special role in the discussions – while pointing out the need for a new leadership – the international community suddenly excluded them from the political process.

THE WAR LOGIC

Political misunderstandings and failures led to a breakdown of relations between UNOSOM and General Aidid, who responded by hardening his position and inciting his supporters to violence. The massacre of twenty-four Pakistani Blue Helmets on 5 June provoked a very firm response from the Security Council and led to attacks by UNOSOM against General Aidid's positions, resulting in a large number of civilian victims. On 12 July a further UN raid turned into a bloodbath, but UNOSOM remained uncompromising and rejected any negotiation.

Against this background of mounting violence, the humanitarian organizations which had managed to operate in relative safety for two years of war in Mogadishu – though at the cost of a number of compromises, mainly the hiring of armed guards – have had to curtail their activities because of increasing insecurity and a growing confusion between the military and the humanitarian roles. More violent incidents are reported daily, guns are back on the streets and there is an upsurge of anti-Western feelings. The UN agencies, pawns in the military operation, have been unable to resume their projects in

Mogadishu, their staff forever being evacuated to Nairobi or trapped in their offices under fire by General Aidid's supporters.

Although this paralysis is confined to the capital and does not call the UN's activities in the other regions of the country into question, it casts a shadow over the future of the international operation in Somalia.

Under its humanitarian trappings, the international operation in Somalia has become increasingly militarized and is now a party to the fighting in Mogadishu. Part of the explanation for the operation going off the rails was its short-term focus, the lack of any clear political aim – a flaw perceptible from the outset. In the absence of any strategy to relaunch political talks and seek a genuine, negotiated solution to the conflict, the military has naturally followed its own logic, and has seemingly become an end in itself. It was all the easier for the military to dominate since it formed the main component of the operation with a budget ten times that of the humanitarian agencies – a paradox in an operation supposedly triggered by the hijacking of 80 per cent of aid by the Somali militia. Rising tension in Mogadishu and the tendency to confuse the humanitarian and the military have not only heightened insecurity but have also considerably reduced the humanitarian organizations' ability to act in the capital. By targeting hospitals and relief compounds, the UN forces behave as if they enjoyed absolute impunity. Not content with stifling the work of aid agencies, the military has ridden roughshod over their basic principles by excessive use of force, which has claimed hundreds of civilian lives. Ordered there to observe, and ensure observance of, the Geneva Conventions, they have cheerfully flouted them, paralysing the aid effort they were supposed to back up initially. Somalia sheds a particularly harsh light on the long-standing contradictions between the military agenda and humanitarian concerns.

Part 2

AN INTERNATIONAL RESPONSE MARKED BY PARADOXES AND AMBIGUITY

11

THE PARADOXES OF ARMED PROTECTION

The number of cases in which relief efforts have been accompanied by armed protection has multiplied in the past three years. Does this mean – as certain politicians have been quick to claim – that conflicts are now beyond the means of conventional – and private – aid organizations? Are we now witnessing an era of 'armed charity'? Or is this nothing more than a pretext used by the major powers to advance their own cause yet again through subterfuge, the real aim being to engage in a new 'policy of mandates' as a prelude to recolonizing the South? Interpretations along these lines are, in actual fact, fragmentary and fairly wide of the mark. It is useful, in order to understand this sensitive issue more clearly, to look at the point of view of the NGOs and to re-examine the problems and paradoxes inherent in the provision of protection for their volunteers.

A NEW CONFLICT ENVIRONMENT

For over twenty years, by travelling to reputedly dangerous far-off places to help civilians or combatants, the NGOs have provided confirmation of an audacious principle – that they are prepared to go where others fear to tread. Consciously or not, they have lent support to the idea that they not only take risks, but the greatest of risks at that. By rejecting any dependence on 'the State', by crossing borders illegally, they ended up convincing themselves that they were the explorers of no-go areas beyond the reach of the legitimate authorities. It did not take much to deduce from this that no one was in charge of such areas and that the NGOs were themselves responsible, by dint of their own efforts, for their own security, something the media were all too ready to proclaim, quite often aided and abetted by ourselves. It was the done thing to trumpet forth that the weary heroes, back from Afghanistan or Angola, had braved unspeakable dangers, something they quite modestly confirmed, leading others to conclude that the NGOs were capable of taking on any kind of danger, anywhere.

But now it is time to drop the pretence. No, the relief areas of the 1980s were not as dangerous as many believed, and during that period protection was accorded *de facto* by the guerrilla movements, for the following three basic reasons.

1 Those guerrilla groups were few in number in any given conflict. The aid workers' 'partners' belonged to well-structured and strong political and military organizations often controlling vast and homogeneous areas (Angola, Eritrea, El Salvador).
2 Against the backdrop of the Cold War each of the belligerents owed allegiance, more or less openly, to one ideological bloc or the other. Respect for human rights and humanitarian principles was one way of achieving the international respectability by which such movements laid great store.
3 These guerrilla fighters had well-organized logistics, usually depending on a kind of 'economic umbilical cord': a safe area along a frontier consisting of refugee camps controlled by one front and receiving supplies from the international community. These 'sanctuaries' provided the fronts with well-ordered war economies and offered refuge to civilians on the other side of the border. A large proportion of the humanitarian relief operations took place in these camps, that is to say outside the combat zones and in regions which all parties – the host countries, the guerrilla fronts and the major powers (via the United Nations) – strove to protect.

All this has changed rapidly over the past few years.

1 Many guerrilla movements are now deprived of their outside support (provided in many cases by the USSR) and are disintegrating rapidly. Where there were once one or two interlocutors, there are now dozens, with such fragmentation leading to the establishment of small and uncontrollable armed bands.
2 Power struggles at world level are nowadays unlikely to be fought via the provision of support for distant guerrilla movements far away in the South. These conflicts are increasingly becoming local – or regional – affairs. Respect for human rights and humanitarian principles is no longer 'in'. Some of the movements (Shining Path, PKK, Khmer Rouge) have even taken a conscious decision to flout such rights and principles in order to shake off the values 'of the North'. As for the armed bands and minor factions, they are out to

establish a reputation for themselves by threatening aid workers rather than protecting them.

3 The main development has been the rapid change in the war economies. The 'sanctuaries' have disappeared (owing to the re-patriation of refugees, as in Cambodia, or a change of attitude in the host country, as in Ethiopia). Wars are moving out of the border areas and spreading into the centres to the effect that the distinction between the rear base, liberated areas and combat zones has disappeared. Civilians can now be found wandering aimlessly in war-torn regions. Southern Sudan, Afghanistan and Angola are countries where this development has taken hold recently.

This unavoidably worsens the situations in which aid workers operate. Forced, in order to get through to the civilians, to enter the very heartland of the battle zones and to move in from the sidelines, they no longer enjoy the protection of the armed movements, which are themselves finding it difficult to preserve their own unity. What is more, these movements no longer have any rear bases along the borders, and are forced to look for supplies within the country itself, usually by preying on the population. Therefore, they no longer usurp humanitarian aid in the way they used to (by diverting it at source) but if need be they will now tear it from the very mouths of its intended recipients by plundering convoys, pillaging and extortion by gangs in the pay of warlords.

Contrary to the idea cultivated all too often, the nature of the conflicts has not changed from being politically and ideologically based in the 1970s and 1980s to being purely economic now. What has happened is that there has been an abrupt breakdown of the war economies, which up till now have been centralized and located in safe areas to the great profit of the guerrilla movements, whose interest lay in protecting the people running those areas.

In this new context the question of protection is becoming central for NGOs. It is at this point that the tenacious myth concerning their total independence falls down, because – unable by their very nature to carry arms themselves – the NGOs must of necessity turn, in order to ensure their own protection, to forces to which they are then beholden. This is not a new issue and many of the ambiguities witnessed in the Cold War era already constituted 'paradoxes of protection'. Nevertheless, things were simpler and the compromises less visible then. If the NGOs were sometimes accused of indirectly funding the war, it was clearly not of their volition. Nowadays, the links between aid and arms are more violent and more blatant, whether it is direct plundering of convoys, wages paid to armed guards or the enforced cohabitation of relief workers with international expeditionary forces.

PROTECTION FROM WITHIN

In order to ensure their protection in this new conflict context, the NGOs have two basic options. The first is the internal option, which consists in trying to find, without any interference from outside, an internal protector within the conflict zone itself. This was the method used throughout the Cold War period, and it must be added that such stable arrangements still exist in some places. A lot of conflicts are still homogeneous in nature; it is possible to approach the two or three warring sides and maintain a neutral profile. Serious, vicious and anarchic conflicts should not be regarded as the general rule for the moment. It is still possible, for example in the mountains of Burma, in Bougainville, Tajikistan, Mauritania, Sri Lanka and Nagorno-Karabakh, to carry out an even-handed humanitarian aid operation spread over a small number of warring factions which continue to give satisfactory protection.

This leaves us with the small number of tragic cases where this balance has broken down. In Somalia, Liberia and Afghanistan it is obvious that the structure of the conflict has changed, no longer involving a stable central government at odds with rebel groups but rather pitting brother against brother and neighbour against neighbour. And this is where aid workers face their first paradox. If, in order to protect themselves, they place themselves under the sphere of influence of a certain faction – assuming they can find one sufficiently strong to guarantee their security – this makes them the enemy of all the others, and what was intended to be their salvation is in reality their undoing. It is almost impossible to avoid this trap because the mere fact of an operation being in a particular geographical area, in a particular zone held by a particular front, is enough to give the impression of support for a certain political group.

It is against this backdrop that the problem of armed guards has to be viewed. The NGOs do not have the means to set up fully-fledged armies to protect their workers. The guards they had in Somalia were only the embodiment of the armed protection of one of the factions. The deterrent effect of such guards stemmed less from the fact that they were armed than from the fact that they belonged to a powerful clan. The natural authority flowing from this, which the weapons merely symbolized, meant the guards did not have to use their arms.

This armed protection is the visible manifestation of the plundering of humanitarian aid by the factions. The insidious tapping of supplies which used to go on in the refugee camps has been replaced by what is tantamount to tribute rendered more openly: payment of guards or 'donation' of some of the aid as recompense for the dominant faction providing protection. The others, the less powerful, are reduced to marauding on the fringes by scavenging on the convoys and attacking those weaker than themselves.

This internal protection is undoubtedly effective. In Somalia, prior to international intervention, relief efforts were still possible and at relatively low human cost. The situation only turns nasty when aid workers – suddenly horrified and sickened by the diversion of supplies they witness – refuse to 'pay up' any more, i.e., no longer accept diversion of a certain – negotiated – amount of relief supplies. In such cases the protective power is placed in jeopardy because it continues to be the target of attacks from the others but is no longer making any 'profit'. The war economy is destabilized.

One should not look, in such internal, confused and fragmented conflicts, at the scale of supply diversion in absolute terms. Rather one should look at the scale it assumes – or assumed – in the 'set-piece' wars involving a 'sanctuary'. The undoubted conclusion would be that there is basically no difference. Intervening in such squalid conflicts means – if the aim is to get to the victims – accepting that an inevitable amount of the aid has to be handed over to the combatants. This is an old paradox, one which is nowadays more visible and which, unquestionably, leaves humanitarian relief efforts open to the charge of being partly responsible for perpetuating such wars. But what is it we want? To save civilians at all costs, or to dry up the conflicts by closing off the combatants' supplies and thus first and foremost condemning all the unarmed victims to further suffering? Those calling for zero diversion of supplies, who are ready – for the sake of drying up the conflict – to leave the civilian population without any help because the factions feed off the aid supplies, are only adding another variant to the long list of violent approaches for dealing with guerrilla forces. Deportation, strategic hamlets, counter-terror against civilians – such methods are based on nothing more than an eternal fantasy of the established powers-that-be, that of draining away the water so that the combatants – who supposedly move among the people like fish in water – will perish. It is clear that this is not compatible with humanitarian principles, and that two aims cannot be achieved in one form of action: that of helping populations and that of ending the war. It has to be accepted that there is a certain contradiction between the two.

FOREIGN PROTECTION

The second context that we have to consider is that in which outside forces – intervening or interposing – undertake to provide protective cover for relief efforts. Here, again, we must distinguish between two types. First, in some countries – usually troublespots left over from the Cold War – we have peacekeeping operations based on agreement between the parties concerned. This is the case, for example, in Cambodia following the Paris Agreements, in El Salvador or Mozambique. These operations give the UN forces an overall political mandate which is usually clear: disarm the factions, organize the repatriation of refugees, get the administration operating again and oversee the holding of free elections. The associated humanitarian aspect poses few problems as it is separate from the political mandate. But there is a need for wariness of future uncertainties in such contexts because these operations can go wrong, as in Angola. If civil war flares up again it is important that the relief organizations are not overtly associated with one side or the other and that they can continue to enjoy relative neutrality. In such operations there must be certain limits with regard to humanitarian and political coordination. Cooperation between relief agencies must be technically effective, but it is not desirable for collusion to arise between the humanitarian and the political players. Apart from this one reservation, such peacekeeping operations cause few problems for aid workers.

But the situation is totally different for the second type of interventions: those in which – without the agreement of the parties concerned – the international community takes it upon itself to protect not the populations, but those who provide them with aid, that is to say, those making relief efforts possible. In Somalia, the argument used to justify the UN Secretary-General's call for the use of force was the scale on which supplies were being diverted from their proper purpose and the alleged blockage of operations. These arguments appear strange now after one year of international presence in that country: the money spent on the allied intervention exceeds by far that lost through the wastage and diversion of aid supplies occurring prior to the international forces' arrival. If the goal really was to save money, then the operation has failed. As for the main argument – that relief operations were being blocked – it has to be admitted that this applied mainly to those of the United Nations. From spring to autumn 1992, when the famine was at its height, the NGOs and the International Committee of the Red Cross saved thousands of lives, and the armed intervention – which came very late in the day – was credited with a success caused in actual fact by the famine itself, which – like a forest fire – burned itself out owing to lack of fuel.

Here, again, we have another of the paradoxes inherent in protection: the need to provide protection was used to justify an action whose real roots lay elsewhere. Protection of relief workers is a pretext pushed forward by governments and international bodies to disguise their real political aims. What were these in the case of Somalia? The craving for media attention of a US president anxious to leave by the front door and have his name emblazoned in history? Probably. Strategic regional interests in a country considered decisive for finalizing the protective ring around the Jerusalem–Riyadh axis? Not very likely. No doubt one of the main reaons was the desire of the UN Secretary-General to avoid disclosure of his organization's bureaucratic failings, made politically visible by the enforced resignation of Mohammed Sahnoun, the only person in a position to breathe fresh life into the search for political solutions while respecting the integrity and complex nature of Somalia. These failings did not take long to manifest themselves technically through the collapse of the second 100-day plan, mainly owing to the UN bigwigs bent on defending their own petty interests and fundamentally incapable of cooperating with one another. The UN proclaimed that protection was impossible and called for outside military help, evidently with the aim of 'ejecting' itself out of the crisis so as not to expose openly its own political and technical shortcomings.

It cannot be denied that difficulties existed prior to the military intervention and that protection was posing a problem. But considering how much more acute the problem has since become, and looking at the cost of the operation, one cannot help but think that the protection of aid workers is an aim largely usurped for the purposes of intervention dictated by quite different intentions. Looking at the situation in former Yugoslavia, the paradox becomes glaringly clear. Nowhere else has the goal of protecting relief workers been more clearly exploited in order to mask other designs, first and foremost that of not really protecting the people themselves. By choosing to ensure the security of food convoys, the governments and the UN have been able to create the impression of a magnificent show of force while at the same time making very sure that their troops did not accomplish what should have been their essential mission, i.e., to firmly stand up to other forces, the very ones responsible for the aggression.

This first paradox residing in outside protection provided by expeditionary forces seems to be congenital. The false moral stance of governments, which is claimed to be a late-twentieth-century phenomenon, is a poor mask for an age-old tendency among politicians – that of hiding their interests under the cover of moralizing declarations. I hold this to be much nearer the truth than the theory mentioned earlier, which is often given greater credence but seems unfounded to me, and which claims that protection of aid workers is a pretext for a new wave of colonialism on the part of a number of countries. Just as the British or the French used the murder of missionaries as a pretext for pacifying and conquering their future colonies, the armies rushing to the aid of relief workers are said to be out to dominate countries which would otherwise escape their embrace. This argument ignores the historical context. Nowadays we are no longer in a phase of expansion, and territory is no longer the decisive criterion of power. The attraction of the South has diminished, the 'historic' lands are shrinking and the great powers are abandoning their entrenched positions. The aim is not to conquer others ravaged by anarchy and war. No, protection of aid workers is more generally a way of doing more or less nothing, soothing the emotions of an agitated public opinion and disguising the abandonment of certain causes, rather than the mantle for a new hegemony.

But in order to assess such intervention measures it is not enough to examine their underlying reasons. We also have to look at what they lead to. Aid workers might be able to live with the fact of their being protected for the wrong reasons if only that protection was adequate.

POLITICO-MILITARY LOGIC VERSUS HUMANITARIAN LOGIC

This is not the case. Quite the contrary, as armed intervention complicates the situation and after an initial relatively calm phase it heightens rather than decreases the danger. This process has been observed in the three major military operations launched with humanitarian aims in the past two years: in Kurdistan, the former Yugoslavia and Somalia. There are two possible situations. In the first of these, the 'humanitarian' armies are themselves belligerents, i.e., directly involved in the conflict. This was the case in Kurdistan. Harassing them and the civilians associated with them is merely a logical continuation of the war. When – as seems almost certainly the case – the Iraqis arrange to have attacks carried out against United Nations agencies in the Kurdish zone, it is merely an extension of their desire to thwart the Americans and to liberate their territory.

Given that the Gulf War allies have moved into the humanitarian field, their Iraqi opponents quite naturally do the same and do not hesitate to target volunteers working there, as was the case with the murder of a member of the French agency, Handicap International, in the spring of 1993.

The second possibility is that the military/humanitarian forces are not *a priori* involved in the conflict. In Yugoslavia and in Somalia, the United Nations peacekeeping forces are a reflection of an international community, which is otherwise all too absent from the local political scene. This sums up the complete ambiguity of this type of operation: action for action's sake, often purely for its media impact, designed to soothe public opinion by 'doing something'. But the decision to move into the humanitarian field is the result of a cruel lack of a political perspective. Protecting humanitarian aid-workers becomes an aim in itself, replacing the age-old need for soldiers to have a political purpose when going to war. This new paradox of protection can be summed up as follows: humanitarian aid permits intervention by armed forces yet gives them no precise political programme.

Clausewitz's theories are not easily dismissed and these 'neutral' expeditionary troops are immediately forced to confront the true nature of the conflict and to become affected by it. As soon as they arrive in the country, peacekeeping troops make the bitter discovery that even if they themselves have no views on the conflict, the belligerents have their conception of what to hope or fear from the international troops. In Somalia, the first United Nations peacekeeping forces were regarded with considerable suspicion by the dominant group (that of General Aidid) which saw itself ready to seize sole power. The interim president Ali Mahdi, by contrast, forcefully demanded international intervention. If General Aidid eventually did welcome the American troops, this was only on the machiavellian principle of making a virtue out of necessity. Thus, even before commencing their operations on Somali soil, the international forces were faced by a complex network of benevolence and hostility.

In former Yugoslavia, while idealistic young UN soldiers continue to see themselves as rescuers as they arrive from Britain and France, those who arrived before them have already made the unpleasant discovery that they are viewed as very far removed from anything humanitarian. Ever since the beginning of the conflict, the Serbs have seen them as a hindrance to their future conquests, the Croats have accused them of 'freezing' the territorial gains made by their enemies, while the Muslims have been vocal in their disappointment at seeing the forces given only a humanitarian mandate.

As their 'humanitarian' trappings are rejected outright, the UN forces are caught in a defensive pattern where the absence of a comprehensive political goal means they respond in an *ad hoc* fashion and they rapidly come to exchange their humanitarian guise for one that is purely and simply military. Originally there to defend humanitarian aid workers, the allied forces soon adopt the goal of defending themselves.

This trend is particularly clear in Somalia where there is an officially identified enemy incarnation of Evil. Getting rid of General Aidid seemed, in the summer of 1993, to have become the new war aim. Focusing in the beginning entirely on the humanitarian aspect – to the point of neglecting such essential steps as disarming and neutralizing the various factions – the international force has embraced an entirely military option – so much so that it has not hesitated to fire missiles at NGO buildings where it felt this was necessary. Is this a U-turn? Far from it. The two phases are linked by the absence of a political plan for Somalia. What should be done with this country and why was there intervention? Failing an underlying motive, the operation is dragged along in the wake of partial, short-term objectives – first humanitarian and then military – dictated by a remorseless logic.

The trend seen in Somalia is also to be found, although in a different guise, in the former Yugoslavia. Whereas in the former the political choice was to find an enemy at all costs where none was apparent, in Bosnia it was the reverse – never to single out an enemy although there was no difficulty in doing so. Deliberately ecumenical, the overriding goal of the intervention was not to be a true inter-vention. Determinedly remaining a humanitarian mission was not the reflection of a pristine purity maintained against all odds but rather of a cynical political decision taken at the outset – to let the Serbs win. This assiduously cultivated impotence is now self-reinforcing. If one prefers not to name the aggressor, circumstances always concur to make this the right decision. The passivity of the UN forces, signifying an acceptance of the crushing of the Bosnians, finally led them to provoke the peacekeeping troops in the hopes that they would react – or rather act. Attacked by those they had the task of defending, the UN forces were forced to the distressing conclusion that all sides were to blame and that impotence was justified.

The paradoxes of protection, wrapped one inside the other like Russian dolls, have transformed the Yugoslav conflict into a series of abdications justified first by the desire to protect the civilian population, then by that of protecting the protectors until finally the paradox peaks with governments justifying their inaction by their fear of compromising the safety of the contingents they have committed. When the victim is sacrificed rather than endangering the appointed protector, one has to concede that the humanitarian/political alliance is full of surprises.

A SCALE OF POLITICAL CLARITY

As we have seen, the association of military and humanitarian activities takes various forms. In essence, these can be classified according to what one might call a scale of political clarity. At the top of the scale come peacekeeping operations arising from international agreements, as in El Salvador, Angola or Cambodia. In such cases, the political aim is clear: to disarm the factions and prepare the country for free elections. As already noted, the humanitarian aspects give rise to few problems – provided over-close and thus dangerous coordination between humanitarian and political actors is avoided.

Next come operations in which the international forces are pursuing war aims which are clear in their own eyes but which cannot be openly stated or which, for one reason or another, they wish to disguise under a cloak of concern. A case in point is Kurdistan. Here, the emergence of a humanitarian dimension reflects a degree of political uncertainty – for example, when the Coalition decided, in March 1991, to stop trying to overthrow Saddam Hussein and to give the Kurds humanitarian aid only. In such circumstances, it is more essential than ever for aid operations to remain independent and neutral, and the NGOs must be careful to eschew all collaboration – let alone integration.

Still further down the scale of political clarity come operations like that in former Yugoslavia, where the major powers have no very clear war aim, but where, if one looks carefully, murky political reasons for this passive attitude can be found – the idea that events should be allowed to take their course in the Balkans so that a stable order can be imposed by force.

Right at the bottom come operations such as in Somalia, where there is absolutely no political rationale and the international community hides behind various masks (humanitarian yesterday, military today) to avoid the question: what are we doing in Somalia?

An interesting point about this scale is that it shows that humanitarian activity is not necessarily incompatible with political or politico-military action by states. When the aims of this action are

clear, it is easy for the aid organizations, while remaining fully independent, to adopt a stance in relation to it, to cooperate or oppose
it, associate themselves with it or keep their distance. The real danger
for humanitarian workers lies in blurred political objectives, in operations without a real aim, in which protection of aid workers – who
never asked for it – becomes a substitute for thinking clearly about
what is to be achieved by armed intervention. All parties in such a
confused situation have a lot to lose. First of all, the politicians and
soldiers, since once the humanitarian phase is over – and often
quickly over – they find themselves in the worst possible predica-
ment, in Sarajevo, Mogadishu or elsewhere: how is force to be used,
when there is no political objective in sight? But the aid organizations,
too, have every reason to fear this unsolicited protection, which
draws them into the ill-directed activities of 'peacekeeping' armies.

The worst aspect is that when the humanitarian side breaks down
in this military/humanitarian association, it is not only the 'official'
humanitarian action, that of the armies and international agencies,
that suffers. In such theatres, all scope for humanitarian action is lost.
Henri Dunant's original concept of a neutral sphere from which the
combatants are excluded is shattered by such operations. The humanitarian sphere is invaded on all sides. The international armies are
the first culprits, with their hotchpotch of political and humanitarian
aims. Their enemies on the ground reply in kind: the Iraqis directly
attack aid workers, whom they equate with the Allies; the Somalis
harass not only the UN forces but also the aid agencies; in Yugoslavia,
red crosses have long been a sniper's target.

Never have so many members of aid organizations paid with their
lives for their commitment as in the last three years, in these theatres
where the military has intervened. This loss of life gives the lie to
those self-satisfied cultivators of public opinion who smugly repeat
that the more aid workers there are, the merrier, and that there is
room for all – the military, national governments and the international
political institutions – in this great and hopeful enterprise. Humanitarian
action, in such difficult and dangerous conditions which are so far
removed from roadside first aid in our own countries, presupposes
impartiality and political independence, and these are qualities which
armies and governments, by their very nature, can never possess.

CONCLUSION

The new environment in which conflicts arise confronts NGOs with
new problems, but they are not insurmountable. At first it seemed,

given the complexity of the situations in Somalia or Yugoslavia, that the NGOs had had their day and the need for protection would mean that armies would come to dominate the humanitarian scene. We must think again. The militarization involved in having operations protected by external forces is a deathtrap and will destroy all humanitarian activity by allowing it to become submerged in a politico-military context in which it cannot survive.

On the contrary, the flexibility and clear thinking of the NGOs has enabled them, in Somalia for example, to maintain a presence throughout the crisis, at a low cost in human terms, and to make sure that essential aid was available. There was certainly considerable misappropriation, but no more than used to occur in the old frontier guerrilla havens, and the cost was certainly less than the enormous expenditure on 'protection' by the American expeditionary force in Somalia. If the major powers wish to intervene in war zones, that is for them to decide, but we should not give them the excuse that they are protecting aid workers. It is difficult enough today for aid workers to protect themselves, without their being the object of the theoretically benevolent and practically detrimental solicitude of politicians at a loss for a policy.

Jean-Christophe Rufin

12

PEACEKEEPING OPERATIONS ABOVE HUMANITARIAN LAW

Since the 1991 Kurdistan intervention, the merits of joint humanitarian and military action have been a subject of debate. Two years later, this 'marriage' has undoubtedly opened the door to a number of United Nations operations (Liberia, Bosnia, Somalia), but there is controversy about their effectiveness from the humanitarian and the military points of view.

At a time when there is renewed discussion about amending the United Nations Charter, it should be remembered that it has not yet been fully applied. Peacekeeping and Blue Helmets are not recent inventions, but a compromise born out of the Cold War and designed to compensate for the inability to use force under Chapter VII of the UN Charter. A Nobel prize has been awarded for these methods, which have been put into practice on a large scale in many conflicts. In the field, however, they suffer from a congenital defect, which is having ever more serious consequences: ambiguity and compromise. The ambiguity of 'keeping the peace' in wartime – a contradiction in terms – has gradually allowed humanitarian operations to breach humanitarian law and military operations to violate the rules of war.

THE PARADOX FACED BY THE UNITED NATIONS: PEACEKEEPING IN TIME OF WAR

The United Nations Charter affirms an ideal: future generations should be spared the tragedy of war. Chapter VI of the Charter sets out practical means of attaining this aim by cooperation and various methods for the pacific settlement of disputes. In Chapter VII, this ideal becomes an ambition. If international peace and security are threatened or breached, the United Nations can use force to restore peace.

For 40 years, the use of the veto made this impossible. However, the United Nations developed a different role, based on Chapter VI. Peacekeeping operations thus involved:

1 a ceasefire signed by the belligerents;
2 an agreement between these parties that the UN should oversee the ceasefire;
3 deployment under the UN flag of lightly armed troops with a mandate to use force in self-defence.

This mechanism is based not on the use of force, but on its deployment as a means of deterrence with the consent of the belligerents. It guarantees the mutual good faith of the parties, and is intended to allow negotiations to resume by halting hostilities. In practice, its only effect has been to freeze conflicts and prevent them from spreading. The emergence of a new consensus in the Security Council has made it possible, in some circumstances, to dispense with the parties' consent to the deployment of troops.

The winter of 1991 was a real turning point. Military action by the international community during and after the Gulf War was based on something other than the agreement of the two parties to the conflict. Two legitimizing concepts then emerged: the threat to international peace and security and humanitarian action.

The threat to peace was effectively countered by the use of force, but without the United Nations' exercising real control. Chapter VII was invoked when the Gulf War was launched, but it could not be used as an operational framework. The United States refused to have the UN Military Staff Committee set up to command the operation. The UN legitimized the war, but did not control it.

In the humanitarian field, force was used in a deterrent mode, in the form of a partial flight ban in conjunction with the deployment on the ground of UN civilian guards. This did not constitute military protection on the ground, but a new and decentralized use of diplomatic protection, which strictly speaking covered only the UN guards, but extended in a very symbolic way to the population by virtue of their physical proximity. However, this protection enabled the UN agencies to carve out a major role for themselves in war zones. Though they did not enjoy the immunity afforded by law to the NGOs, they have managed to substitute this extended form of diplomatic protection. Set up to give expression to cooperation between sovereign states, these organizations were neither designed, nor prepared, to intervene in conflicts.

Humanitarian law seeks to minimize the strategic value of aid for the victims so that the presence of aid workers will be tolerated amid the hostilities. Its aim is to save as many people as possible from the suffering and destruction of war. Such law is not imposed, but spread by contact. Peacekeeping and peacemaking, by contrast, require the permanent use of compromise and the skilful juggling of dialogue and deterrent or offensive force. The new UN intervention derived rather from new concepts, such as safe havens, humanitarian cease-fires and peace corridors. These 'bubbles of peace', artificially created in the midst of conflict, are ineffective in preventing fighting. Worse, this new type of humanitarian action protects the providers of aid and their convoys rather than the victims.

The full absurdity of this shift in approach became apparent in the former Yugoslavia. By deploying its troops there, the UN, following in the footsteps of the EC, endorsed hybrid forms of intervention. This is no longer peacekeeping, since the warring parties cannot agree on the terms of peace. Such international intervention derives its authority not from the use of force, but from the quality of its humanitarian good intentions. As early as May 1992, the United Nations was assert-ing that it was not possible to undertake military operations in Bosnia-Herzegovina. The objective of the international intervention would therefore be more modest: to promote ceasefires, to observe the daily ceasefire violations (Resolution 749, 1992) and to protect aid convoys (Resolution 776, 1992). Meanwhile, Resolution 771 condemned the failure to respect the humanitarian obligations deriving from the Geneva Conventions. However, no decision was ever taken on the means necessary to put a stop to these violations. As a result, the deployment of UN troops did not have the anticipated deterrent effect. The UN force was unable to do more than record the violation of these principles and prohibitions.

Since UN troops are not authorized to use force, it is always difficult to say whether the soldiers are protecting the aid workers or the other way round. What is clear is that both have become targets as each hides behind the other's skirts. It is well known that convoys are held up, that there is no access to detention camps and that the slightest agreement has to be paid for in terms of corruption, compromising of principles and allowing war criminals to go unpunished. It is also common knowledge that since the deployment of United Nations forces in the former Yugoslavia, every decision is carefully weighed up against the possible implications for the safety of the international troops. The old peacekeeping approach, which implies separating the combatants, has placed the international troops in an untenable position where they are, in effect, hostages. The troops are not only – as a matter of policy – lightly armed but also encircled. In this situation, the only non-violent barter currency is humanitarian aid. In this military, political and humanitarian horse-trading, UN operations seriously undermine the fundamental principles of humanitarian law, although these operations are still vital and many hopes are pinned on them. It is therefore important that there be a return to a more principled stance.

UN PERVERSITY: AID OPERATIONS WHICH VIOLATE HUMANITARIAN LAW

The Geneva Conventions and their additional protocols represent a comprehensive and pragmatic system which maintains a constant balance between military imperatives and the scope for limiting unnecessary suffering and destruction. Under cover of a new, idealistic 'humanitarian mania', the UN's activities depart radically from this strict framework for humanitarian action.

The main achievement of humanitarian law lies in the protection afforded to non-combatants: civilian property and objectives may not be attacked. The UN resolutions adopted in connection with the flight of the Kurds and the Yugoslav and Somali conflicts all refer to the protection of aid convoys – a new doctrine in humanitarian action – while not one mentions the protection of the victims. The civilian population is regarded solely as the recipient of aid, which is lavishly provided with the best of intentions, even if it never reaches its intended target. Preoccupation with logistics eclipses concern for human beings, as if soap or milk powder could prevent bombs from falling on hospitals, or generosity could offer protection against murder and expulsion.

The Geneva Conventions prescribe different roles for governments and NGOs. Governments must comply and ensure compliance with humanitarian law and have the duty to use all necessary means to halt serious violations of it. The role of NGOs is to provide independent and unconditional help to victims, with the support of governments.

Today, the UN, with its various institutions, is at the forefront of aid operations, which it conducts in parallel with a process of politico-military negotiation. But how can the pursuit of peace fail to stifle the demand for justice? Negotiation with criminals always presupposes that they will be allowed to escape punishment. When the reports of the UN Commission on Human Rights identify the guilty parties in the Yugoslav conflict, the Security Council rushes to set up a new body to investigate whether the existence of these crimes can be substantiated. Where is there a sphere free from all strategic considerations in which the NGOs can pursue their humanitarian activity?

The Geneva Conventions assert that prisoners should be freed unilaterally and unconditionally. But there is always someone among the representatives of the international community who is prepared to organize the exchange of a group of prisoners of war for an equivalent number of civilian hostages. For almost a year now, no prisoners have been freed in the former Yugoslavia through the good offices of the ICRC, because there was always a 'humanitarian' broker with a better offer.

Humanitarian law in the broadest sense of the term affirms the principle that refugees should not be turned back as central to the protection of individuals in times of crisis. In the former Yugoslavia, UNPROFOR has been accused of opposing access by refugees to the security zones it controlled. This was of course in line with a political assurance given to the warring parties, which the United Nations had to honour. But it is cause for concern that this assurance should have led to the decision to turn back people seeking refuge. This attitude reflects a deep-seated ignorance of legal principles and humanitarian duties. In adhering to the terms of its mandate, UNPROFOR gave greater weight to a political undertaking than to a categorical legal obligation. Humanitarian law has the mandatory force of international conventions and always takes precedence over obligations prescribed by UN resolutions. The UN's failure to reaffirm the precedence of humanitarian law over the constraints of a peacekeeping, or peacemaking, mandate has serious consequences.

In Liberia, the regional peacekeeping force carried this paradox to its logical conclusion by twice destroying aid convoys. Whatever the official explanations, what clearly emerges is the conflict between peacekeeping operations and humanitarian assistance: according to the commanders of the West African force, aid operations were delaying the 'final victory' of the peacekeepers. Does this mean that a just war is the best means of putting a stop to the suffering caused by an unjust war? If this argument were to prevail, we would have to start all over again to recreate a sphere for humanitarian action. Such action does not seek to make peace or win wars but to introduce a little humanity in the midst of violence.

UN IMPUNITY: MILITARY OPERATIONS WHICH VIOLATE THE LAWS OF WAR

The way in which international military operations developed found the UN unprepared in two respects: operational organization and strategic legality. Since the Military Staff Committee provided for by the Charter has not been set up, command of UN operations in the field is always a compromise between national command structures, which may or may not work well together. The consequences are apparent at several levels. Different national contingents have their own interpretations of the mandate and it is thus always difficult to make an overall assessment and critique of operations. Everyone and no one is responsible for controlling the UN forces. There is no common code of military discipline within the UN, no military police with responsibility for investigating abuses by military personnel, no authority to punish the guilty and compensate their victims. Self-criticism goes no further than expressions of regret at abuses committed by some less well-organized contingents. But there is very limited respect for authority and discipline in the national contingents, since in any case the orders come from the UN.

Today, the UN goes on the military offensive, but without accepting its status as a belligerent subject to the laws of war. Does it regard itself as above the law? Are no holds barred as long as one's purpose is to restore peace, to overthrow oppressors and cut the cost to the international taxpayer? The laws governing armed conflict impose strict limits on the use of force, irrespective of the cause at stake or the adversary. In Liberia, aid convoys are attacked by a regional force acting under the authority of the UN Security Council. In Somalia, the increasingly open dissension between the national contingents confirms the NGOs' accusations that humanitarian law is being breached by the UN forces. UN attacks are not accompanied by the precautions and early warnings required to protect civilians and civilian premises. Civilian districts are bombarded without warning and without prior evacuation. Hospitals are attacked, access to medical care is impeded and medical assistance prevented.

It is no exaggeration to say that international policing operations are in a dangerous state of flux. Their legality must be strengthened and anchored in humanitarian law, which applies to all and which it is their function to uphold. What is worrying is that it has not yet been possible to define what clearly constitutes a sufficient threat to peace and international security to justify armed intervention. For the present, the case of Yugoslavia demonstrates that flagrant and massive violations of humanitarian law is seen as a threat to the peace and security of no one but the victims.

Françoise Bouchet-Saulnier

13

THE HUMAN RIGHTS CHALLENGE TO SOVEREIGNTY

Since the Treaty of Westphalia in 1648, the principle that countries are sovereign states, separate and equal, has been the main tenet of international relations. As if the higher value of human rights had not become established in the meantime, the United Nations' Charter of 1945 confirmed the inviolability of the principle that every ruler is master in his own house, whatever he does. Although it has been realized for centuries that the doctrine of sovereignty is, in practice, more an ideal than a reality, only recently – since the 1991 Gulf War against Iraq, to be precise – has this doctrine obviously been called into question, or, rather, become totally obsolete, since it ceased to apply to countries ostracized by the international community at the instigation of the major powers.

To be fair, this erosion of sovereignty seems to affect both northern and southern countries, but in the former case it has taken the form of voluntary, 'sovereign' concessions, to which countries have consented for the sake of closer regional ties or as a result of the kind of 'private sovereignty' exercised by London or Wall Street foreign exchange dealers when they bring western currencies to their knees. In the southern countries, however, and in recent years in eastern ones as well, the loss of sovereignty has not been voluntary, and has had little to do with market forces or with a proper balance between interdependent states. Where they are concerned, the refusal to recognize sovereignty comes increasingly from other, Western states which, generally – but not always – under the cloak of the United Nations, claim the so-called 'right to interfere', having decided either that the state in question does not exist any more and has consequently lost its sovereignty (Somalia), or that it is exercising its sovereignty in a criminal fashion (Iraq). Moreover, to place the whole process beyond criticism, this right to interfere is almost always attributed to the desire to defend human rights.

SOVEREIGNTY CURTAILED VOLUNTARILY OR BY FORCE

While there can be no doubt about the nobility of the alleged motives, the manner of putting them into practice may be a stumbling block to the progress that human rights and, above all, the basic right to life have made over the centuries. In its modern version, the history of human rights began with the French Revolution which, paradoxically, instituted the rights of 'citizens', in the abstract, but also introduced the forced conscription of those same flesh-and-blood human beings. Since the lives of conscripts, of which there was an almost infinite supply, were held much more cheaply than the lives of the *ancien régime* mercenaries, who were expensive to recruit, wars became very much more murderous than when they had to all intents and purposes been a matter of besieging towns and cities. And it was shortly after the revolutionary or nationalist massacres which marked the heyday of the principle of national sovereignty that the situation became so disgraceful that the idea of humanitarian conventions took root in the mind of Henri Dunant at the Battle of Solferino in 1859. Nation-states would sign these conventions voluntarily in order to 'recivilize' their armed conflicts. We shall skip the later details: the setting up of the International Committee of the Red Cross, the first Geneva Convention of 1864, the Hague Convention and Rules of 1899 and 1907 and the four Geneva Conventions of 1949 with the two 1977 additional protocols. The salient feature of the humanitarian conventions is scrupulous respect for national sovereignty to the extent that they are legally binding only if they have been accepted and signed (non-signatories, such as the Soviet Union during the Second World War, are not covered). Geneva-style humanitarianism is noteworthy for referring in its first phase only to wounded and sick members of the armed forces or prisoners. It was not extended until 1949 to civilian victims or non-uniformed combatants in internal conflicts – civil wars, guerrilla and resistance movements. While this was a major extension of protection, it still applied only to foreign or civil wars – in short, to the effects of belligerency in a spirit of reciprocity on the part of the warring parties. It has *not* affected the cornerstone of the sovereignty of every state, i.e., the way in which that sovereignty is exercised, with or without respect for the universal rights which all those subject to the state's authority ought to have enjoyed. Governments and even blood-soaked tyrants have continued to enjoy a free hand on their own territory.

The current logic of restrictions on national sovereignty imposed in the name of the universal values of respect for individuals (as well as, nowadays, for nature or the environment) is another matter. Since 1945, this logic has found expression, though to no great effect, in Chapter VII of the UN Charter, which in theory gives the United Nations the power to use force against countries posing a threat to international peace and security. American intervention in Korea, however, was simply a reflection of power politics, and the main aim of the 1960 UN intervention in Katanga was to save the lives of Europeans in danger. Two resolutions of the UN General Assembly, adopted in 1970 and 1981 under pressure from former colonies and from communist states, consistently opposed to any interference in their internal affairs, even in order to defend human rights, confirmed in practice the inviolability of the principle of sovereignty.

It was not until East–West relations began to improve that, on the initiative of France, the opposite, but as yet tentative, principle of intervention made its appearance in the two resolutions of 8 December 1988 and 14 December 1990. One refers to humanitarian assistance granted – in a secondary capacity only, when the country concerned cannot cope alone – in the case of a natural catastrophe or similar disaster, and the other provides for the opening up of humanitarian corridors in times of war. It was this latter resolution which was applied to bring help to the Croatian city of Dubrovnik at the end of 1991 – although it was not applied in the case of Vukovar. Even before that, however, it was clear that Security Council Resolution 688 of 5 April 1991 had marked the turning point towards intervention on a totally different scale, when the Iraqi Government was made to grant free access to international aid for the oppressed Kurds.

INTERVENTION AS AN OPTIONAL EXTRA?

The first part of this book has shown that, more generally, humanitarian operations of all kinds have in recent years been prompted by factors which ultimately had very little to do with the depth of human suffering. In other words, even though the defence of human rights or the most basic concern for people's survival may have provided some justification for taking action, there has been other motivation of a political kind. Have the industrialized countries which have intervened cared as much about the effectiveness of their actions from the humanitarian point of view as about obtaining a seal of approval from the world at large or from public opinion at home?

There are and always have been human disasters which have not led to any official action on the part of the United Nations or of the major powers: Biafra and, today, Afghanistan and southern Sudan.

There are others, just as terrible, where it appeared to be sufficient to delegate action to a regional organization with very few resources – in particular in Liberia, under the cloak of the West African peace-keeping forces, or others in which a world power running out of steam, namely Russia, is allowed freedom of action around its own borders, especially in the Caucasus and Tajikistan. At the same time, there are cases where action takes the form of UN operations which are militarized to a greater or lesser extent and which in fact aim solely to clean up the after-effects of the East–West conflict: Angola and Cambodia since 1991, Nicaragua in 1989–90 and even El Salvador in 1991–2. The roll-call ends for the moment with armed emergency 'humanitarian' intervention, initially the Somalia operation legitimized by Council Resolution 794 of 3 December 1992 and subsequently two separate UN operations in Croatia and Bosnia, and, less openly, in the no-fly zones imposed on the Iraqi air force on its own national territory.

Why have these operations taken place, or failed to take place, and why in one form rather than another? In greatly simplified terms, it would seem that they initially arose from the void left by the implosion of the international system which until that point had been locked in the East–West confrontation, and that they were born of the changing spirit of the times in the prosperous West. Now that the early phase of 1988–91 is over and the process has become established, it would appear that one state intervenes in the affairs of another (or of a state declared non-existent) as part of the competition between advanced countries anxious to maintain their footholds on humanitarian/military territory. A more important cause has been the recent need to justify maintaining armed forces now that the serious risk of an East–West confrontation has evaporated.

Admittedly, Western diplomats, aided by the Helsinki negotiations, kept up the constant pressure about human rights from the start of the 1970s to the fall of the Berlin Wall, but they touted the Helsinki Agreements in regard to human rights merely to embarrass the Soviet Union. It would have been difficult to invoke human rights to justify arms supplies to the Afghan rebels or CIA support for the anti-Sandinista resistance movement in Nicaragua or American military intervention in Grenada in 1983 not to mention France's collusion with African dictators. The shameful events in Cambodia, in particular, when the Western powers defended the 'legitimate' sovereignty of the Khmer Rouge solely in order to thwart Vietnam, the Soviet Union's loyal ally, made it crystal clear how indifferent they were to human rights.

And so nothing changed until 1989–90, when this purely Platonic debate on human rights – in Eastern Europe – lost its strategic importance. At the same time, however, it was important to the major democracies to continue to affirm their superiority where values were concerned, at least *vis-à-vis* the southern countries, since the East European countries had greater need of money than of advice. They therefore pushed the button marked 'democratization'. Unfortunately, since post-communist democratic processes, like those in Africa or even Latin America, sometimes tended to get bogged down, they just as quickly had to return to the theme of human rights, only this time enshrining it in a minimalist doctrine of emergency aid coupled with a maximalist obligation to interfere in order to bring that aid. This new outlook also appeared to coincide perfectly with the mood of the times in the prosperous West, where activists had, in effect, given up their development credo, losing all belief in the possibility of helping the Third World to escape its poverty-ridden existence, henceforth regarded with a kind of culturally-driven fatalism. Moreover, public opinion in the democratic countries displayed growing intolerance towards their 'un-Western' immigrants. And so the practice of intervention to defend values which had become hard to find at home came just at the right moment.

All this, of course, simply explains how the reversal of attitudes originally came about. What we have to consider now is humanitarian intervention observed as events unfold. At this level, cost/benefit calculations (covert, of course) appear to underlie the noble motives trumpeted abroad. But the problem for anyone trying to bring it to the world's attention is that these calculations have been befogged by the fact that no strategic interests are any longer at stake in most cases, with the exception of Iraq as a theatre for intervention and the UN as an actor on the international stage. Iraq is an incontrovertible case, since everyone is well aware that Operation Provide Comfort in Kurdistan was a useful way of disguising the partial failure of the Gulf War, which could not get rid of Saddam Hussein for fear of disturbing the balance in the Gulf region. Neither is there any doubt about the United Nations, whose prestige has been temporarily bolstered by that earned by its Blue Helmets. But what reasons lie behind other operations, where the stakes are less readily apparent, or behind operations yet to take place? Maybe we should remember the philosopher de Mandeville's Fable of the Bees.

DE MANDEVILLE'S FABLE

In the Fable of the Bees, de Mandeville argued that even actions prompted by dubious motives could produce public benefits. An obvious case in point was the humanitarian Operation Provide Comfort in Iraq, though this operation was secondary to military action and disguised the fact that that action had not been brought to a successful conclusion. It was even more the case with the combined military/humanitarian Operation Restore Hope launched in Somalia in December 1992. There were fears at the time, since proven to have been well-founded, that this would endanger humanitarian activities. Maybe President Bush was aware of the risk and, since Bill Clinton had already been elected, he did not even have the excuse of a warlike gesture to assist in his re-election campaign. Moreover, Somalia was no longer (unlike Iraq) of strategic importance to the United States: it was only an exercise ground where the Americans' patriotic fervour, always of the most humanitarian and catholic kind, could be boosted. But even if this playing to the gallery hampered the private aid agencies and left innocent victims to be cared for by the doctors from Europe, it also enabled thousands of tons of food supplies to be delivered, saving a great number of lives. Consequently, is the problem not, rather, that intervention which fails to materialize, as in southern Sudan, for a *raison d'état* is just as questionable as those examples invoked above? Or, again, are operations such as those in Bosnia which use humanitarian gestures as an excuse for military inaction explicitly justified by the excessive cost of effective armed action? The chosen venue must thus lend itself to spectacular forms of action which prove effective in the short term or must be one in which the stakes, as well as the cost, are high, as in the Gulf.

What are human rights worth today? First, since the Gulf War the 'defence of human rights' has become the sticker to be placed on any diplomatic or military action by the West, so much so that it tends to conceal other motives, temporarily, at least.

Second, in most other cases it is the vacuum created by the crumbling away of the sovereignty of an increasing number of southern and eastern countries which has led, or rather drawn, some countries to intervene on these new 'humanitarian' grounds, especially in Somalia, Liberia, the former Yugoslavia or the southern frontiers of Russia.

Third, it would seem that these power vacuums stimulate rivalry between developed countries eager to plunge in and find a role for their Blue Helmets, as witness the recent difference of opinion between

France and Australia over the training of armed forces in Cambodia. Apart from anything else, armed humanitarianism looks like giving a new lease of life to military authorities who have suddenly turned to spearheading a universal philanthropic movement.

Finally, the most optimistic hypothesis could be that intervention operations, so virtuously dedicated to human rights, may prove beneficial in retrospect. After all, when Britain arrogantly asserted its right to stop and search foreign ships on the pretext of combating slavery, its main objective was to consolidate its world supremacy. Nevertheless, these inspections sounded the death-knell of slave-trading and slavery. It may well be, therefore, that, for all its ambiguities and contradictions, intervention for the sake of defending human rights will, against all expectations, enhance the dignity of mankind and begin to unlock the doors imprisoning each country in the fortress of its own sovereignty.

Guy Hermet

14

HEALTH-CARE RECONSTRUCTION
The lost agenda

In countries undergoing reconstruction, international assistance can be of central importance to the health system. The ethical and human considerations are unquestionable and no state in difficulty would turn down an offer to help rebuild its health-care system. Similarly, no donor country would question the need for or the advisability of such assistance. Any government would have to take action in this area, if only to become more popular with its people or to command more respect from donor countries. Demonstrating an interest in health problems is a good way of winning the approval of donor countries for which 'health indicators' are criteria which allow a judgement to be made as to whether or not a state is behaving responsibly, all the more so when the state in question is a young and unstable regime emerging from a crisis which has attracted international attention.

The rebuilding of health-care systems is therefore, from the political point of view, an opportunity for those concerned to offer evidence of their legitimacy. To take a cynical view, it could be seen as a clever political marketing ploy, irrespective of the extent to which the system has to be rehabilitated.

While the aim of rehabilitating health-care systems is clearly a laudable one, there remains the question of the provisions made by the international community to achieve it. The deficiencies in meeting that aim are sometimes evidence of a lack of real commitment after a fine flurry of public statements of good intentions. Another factor here is accountability. In other words, what expertise, what skills are really deployed for the rehabilitation of those health-care systems?

For example, in mid-1992, shortly after its arrival in Cambodia, the United Nations Transitional Authority in Cambodia (UNTAC) appointed a director for rehabilitation; this greatly encouraged the different organizations working in the health field. The largest UN operation ever mounted could draw on vast resources to launch a large-scale reconstruction of a health-care system.

The different relief agencies which had been active in increasing numbers in Cambodia since the end of the 1980s had already started on this immense task, through a series of more or less coordinated actions. They had thus managed to provide a semblance of health cover which, however, only exposed more clearly the need for action which would be more comprehensive, more conclusive and founded on a sound policy. Their hopes were soon disappointed.

WHEN SHOULD RECONSTRUCTION BEGIN?

The first difficulty lies in determining when the rehabilitation phase should begin. In other words, at what point should actions cease to be a mere palliative and should consideration be given to longer-term objectives? Experience shows that there is no real hiatus between the rebuilding phase and what came before. However, the answer to the question is not without interest since a faulty assessment of the situation can lead to delays and serious setbacks.

The difficulty with choosing the right moment and adapting programmes to the local context was especially evident in Somalia. As early as the beginning of 1993, with the country still ravaged by famine and in a state of complete political chaos, the representatives of the main international medical organizations (UNICEF, WHO), relying solely on the promises of the Operation Restore Hope, announced the launch of complex health programmes such as the 'extended vaccination programme', the anti-tuberculosis programme and the re-establishment of the national programme of health information. These financially and technically demanding programmes required operational health-care structures, competent and motivated personnel and a level of security ensuring free movement and reliable communications, conditions which even now have not been met. This being the case, should the announcement be seen merely as an adjunct to the armed intervention or was it simply evidence of complete ignorance of the actual situation in the country? In any event the programmes had very great difficulty in getting off the ground and were finally shelved.

A good evaluation is therefore needed from the outset, especially because in countries which are being 'reconstructed', the pre-war systems have not entirely disappeared. It is never possible to start with a clean slate. Instead, it will be found that grafts will have been added to the original system, adjustments made and provisional health-care structures cobbled together. There is an overlapping of these different systems and, more importantly, the people involved remain when the new 'era' is inaugurated. Thus in Cambodia the problem was to know what model should serve as the basis for rehabilitation. It is obvious that any such system is influenced by the policy adopted by the previous regime and in periods of transition decisions about new directions require a delicate touch.

The Cambodian health-care system in 1992 was based directly on the very decentralized Vietnamese model, which relied on a large network of village dispensaries. However, there were also many more hospitals than were needed in the capital, Phnom Penh, relics of the 1960s abandoned for lack of funds. The picture was of a multitude of health-care structures at different levels, the only common feature being their run-down condition. There was also the pressing question of matching human resources to the health policy options. As a result of the Khmer Rouge massacres, which had taken a heavy toll among medical staff, the authorities after 1979 had introduced emergency training programmes in order to create a new generation of health-care personnel as soon as possible. Training for an ordinary nurse consisted of a course of barely twelve months after leaving primary school. This policy made it possible in ten years to 'produce' five times as many nurses as the country had ever had in the past, even in peacetime. The down side of this very generous level of staffing was the very low level of qualification of all health-care professionals. For example, hospital directors have no managerial skills since they have never been required to manage anything in the past; all decisions were in fact taken by a 'people's committee' which was answerable not to the Ministry of Health but to the Ministry of the Interior and to the Party.

In such a situation, what rehabilitation programme can be implemented and, moreover, what organizational model can be used as a benchmark? What international authority can draw up a balance sheet and propose solutions? What political power is in a position to take the necessary decisions and determine priorities when all the players are convinced that a major political change is imminent and there is as yet no government, only a provisional administration? In Cambodia it seems that all these questions have by and large not been answered. The lack of a clearly defined model or overall plan, the absence of decisions about matters concerning the allocation and the function of health-care structures, about the number and the qualification of medical personnel and about the financing and management system for those structures make the task of reconstruction extremely difficult and call into question the ability of the international community to play an effective part in the process.

REHABILITATION, A CLEARLY DEFINED STAGE IN AN EMERGENCY SITUATION

The rehabilitation period is one stage in the recovery process that requires different methods from those used in an emergency situation, where all available resources are directed towards the victims with the aim of saving as many lives as possible – which often justifies large-scale aid from other countries. In rehabilitation the objective should be the gradual strengthening of the existing structures, and this means recognizing the central importance of those playing a part in the country's health-care system: doctors, hospital directors, nurses, etc.

In Cambodia, according to the latest figures from the Ministry of Health, there are more than 22,000 public service salaried health professionals, including an incredible number of 6,000 trained by aid groups in refugee camps in Thailand between 1979 and 1993. Doctors and nurses in Cambodia are poorly paid and they have gradually devised a system of remuneration in which earnings from the lucrative private sector are an important supplement to their public sector pay. This is a natural reaction in many poor countries to enable health-care personnel and their families to make ends meet. Nowadays they all have a private practice and in addition there are innumerable unofficial practitioners – retired nurses, pseudo-nurses trained under Pol Pot or, most of them, real quacks. As a result, the distinction between public hospital and private practice is increasingly blurred, to the effect that no treatment can be guaranteed without payment.

Health-care rehabilitation should therefore focus on re-establishing a public health system, bringing hospitals back into the public sector, providing treatment for the poor, for lepers and those with tuberculosis, and ensuring a place again for preventive medicine, a service never provided for in the private sector. Support from the workforce for such a return to a public health service requires delicate negotiations covering matters such as pay prospects, job motivation, working conditions and equipment. If the rehabilitation of the national army involves identifying soldiers and getting them back to barracks so as to distinguish them from the real bandits, this could serve as an analogy for the problem of rehabilitating health-care staff. The international players, foremost amongst them the special agencies of the United Nations, have a serious responsibility in this area.

These are the objectives which all the medical organizations working in Cambodia (ICRC, NGOs and the national Red Cross societies) had for some years been trying to achieve in order to restore normal working conditions and reinstate the public sector to the position it had previously enjoyed. This was a task requiring a patient and sensitive approach, which should have led to defining the objectives of the rebuilding effort through a dialogue with the parties concerned. Paradoxically, this work was compromised by UNTAC when, in each military region, it set up field hospitals – segregated units managed exclusively by foreign personnel. Of course, rehabilitation was not now the purpose of the exercise. These field hospitals were first aid posts for any of the 15,000 soldiers in the United Nations contingent. Serious problems arose when UNTAC recruited Cambodian supervisory personnel to meet its own operational needs. Several hundred people, able to speak either English or French, were 'seconded' from the health and education sectors, with a pay more than ten times their official salary. District hospitals lost their supervisory staff, with the result that the hospital service, already very poor, deteriorated even further. In addition, many UNTAC army doctors, clearly for humanitarian reasons, began to provide treatment for the civilian population. Although this could be justified in some isolated areas, it more often than not created serious problems by diverting the population from hospitals which, with the assistance of NGOs, had begun to treat patients again. There was no reason whatsoever to think that this medical initiative – the creation by UNTAC of a parallel system prompted only by internal requirements – would in any way help rebuild the national system.

FUNDING CAPACITY TO MATCH AMBITIONS

Reconstruction schemes must of necessity form part of a medium and long-term strategy, which calls for a long-term financial commitment on the part of international donors. At first, the promised funds are often impressive as donors pledge appropriately large sums to demonstrate their commitment. When a particular problem is in the news, they are also concerned that their aid should be clearly visible.

In June 1992 a major conference of aid donors to Cambodia was held in Tokyo. The delegates came back full of enthusiasm: the international community had offered 880 million dollars, well above the estimated requirement of 600 million for priority needs. Later on it became clear that in the rush to announce the provision of large reconstruction funds, they had misinterpreted the donors' subtle terminology to distinguish between funds that are promised, vaguely planned or actually committed. A year later, only 212 million had actually been paid and 41 million spent in various ways. So the funds actually available for rehabilitation were still a rare if not non-existent commodity, and they were paradoxically more difficult for the NGOs to get at after the arrival of UNTAC. Capital expenditure usuallly poses few problems because it is visible, but the servicing costs, so essential for maintaining the new systems, are rarely given sufficient consideration. The sums involved in reconstruction programmes are often large, but specialists are still surprised by the lack of flexibility in using them, which sometimes leads to the impression that funds are being wasted.

Salaries represent the largest item in a public finance budget in developing countries and Cambodia, with its 22,000 health workers, is no exception to the rule. Average salaries range from eight to twelve dollars, although nearly a hundred would be needed to live decently; but the Ministry of Health is poorly funded. There was a recurring rumour, in the hospitals, that 'UNTAC is going to pay next month's salaries'. But of course it never happened, partly for reasons of neutrality – aid would have been equivalent to support for the government in office – and partly because the donors were perplexed by the plethora of staff. Of course there were grounds for doubt, but isn't the situation simply the result of a problem recognized at a higher level and left unsolved because of a gap in the decision-making machinery? What hope is there for a new, improved health policy which fails to address the central question of pay?

Conversely, other budget items which may seem large on a national scale turn out to be derisory in relation to the UN's operating expenditure. For example, the total annual expenditure on drugs and renewable medical equipment was estimated at 7.5 million dollars for all hospitals and dispensaries in the country. The cost of the whole operation for restoring peace was nearly two billion dollars – so the cost of a single day of peacekeeping would amply cover a whole year's worth of drugs for the whole country! This disparity became even clearer when Cambodian staff came desperately pleading for the one million dollars needed to supply national anti-TB treatment for a year. In Cambodia TB is at world record levels, with an estimated 20,000 new sufferers per year and 10,000 fatalities. The supply of medication for the programme had dried up and almost all treatment had to be discontinued. Bearing in mind that the daily *per diem* allowance paid to UN personnel on top of their salary is 150 dollars, and that it would have been enough for the 7,000 administrators and UN police to give up one day's *per diem* to prevent these deaths, it is not hard to imagine the perplexity of Ministry of Health staff when the UNTAC representative told them at a special emergency meeting that there was no money available for this purpose.

COORDINATION AND PARTNERSHIP – KEY CONCEPTS FOR REHABILITATION

The problem of the supply of medicines, so vital to any health-care system, provides a good illustration of the difficulty of coordinating a scheme to achieve a predefined objective.In January 1991, due to the failure of COMECON and the introduction of the free market, the supply of drugs in the public sector collapsed completely in Cambodia. Imports which had been estimated at 5.5 million dollars in 1990 fell to less than one million when the USSR made it clear to its partners that in future the bills would have to be paid in dollars. As a result most hospitals were paralysed. This drastic shortage was very slightly offset by humanitarian aid in the form of kits provided by UNICEF and direct donations of medicines mainly by non-governmental and Red Cross organizations. The relaunching of a national system for the supply of drugs was declared a priority in 1992 and led to the creation of a major national project involving WHO, UNICEF and various NGOs. A list of requirements was drawn up and potential donors were sought.

At the Tokyo Conference, instructions had been given to NGOs not to make individual requests to the various donors in future, as the conference provided an opportunity to obtain an overview of the various requirements which could be met by concerted coordination of all the donors wishing to come to the aid of the Cambodian people working their way towards peace under the UN umbrella. As already shown, all these laudable efforts to coordinate fund-raising produced only a very meagre result. And on the other hand, no provision had been made for expenditure. Serious differences emerged between the United Nations and other aid groups, leading to fights as bitter as the money was scarce. UNTAC proposed using the funds earmarked for buying medicines to carry out a major operation distributing medical kits to all the villages in the country. Given that people were starting to query the efficiency of the United Nations, this might have been a vote-winning ploy to bolster the peace process. Whatever the reason, this sprinkling of aid, unrelated to concerns for health and above all for the re-establishment of the system, would have gravely prejudiced the long-term work undertaken by humanitarian organizations. Even more seriously, such a wide distribution operation would have paralysed the national health care system even further, by using up the scant resources available. As a result there was serious opposition to the project and even UNICEF was completely against it, illustrating yet another of the many differences of opinion between the traditional UN agencies and UNTAC. The idea of coordination stayed on the drawing board, powerless in the face of the interests in play. In the end the project was cancelled and the money was given to the aid agencies.

As we have seen, the difference between a rehabilitation strategy and an emergency strategy is that rehabilitation is concerned not only with the impact on the people affected but also with the re-establishment of a system and its traditional players. That is why it is essential to develop partnerships with all the parties involved. Our experience in Cambodia demonstrates yet again that the unwieldiness, power and arrogance of the UN machine deployed in these major operations is incompatible with the need to take advantage of the know-how of people with long experience in the field. Not only were Cambodia's health professionals completely disregarded – even international NGOs were virtually ignored by UNTAC, at least initially. It was not until the fifth month of effective UN presence that a first technical meeting was convened by its representative, Mr Akashi, who suddenly wanted to ask the opinion of the NGOs involved in the health sector, in some cases already for several years and on a large scale. This meeting, which had no definite agenda and was supposed to be informal, soon degenerated into confrontation and signalled a transition in UNTAC's attitude to NGOs from one of total disregard to one of mistrust. It was only much later, at the beginning of 1993, and in view of UNTAC's increasing unpopularity in the country, that the officials responsible issued a document under the heading of the 'Civic Action' Programme, advising their local officials to place their huge logistic resources at the disposal of the NGOs, trying to restore their image by associating themselves with the humanitarian operations carried out by the NGOs in direct contact with the population. Thus began a new stage in our collaboration which, despite the pitiful funds provided, allowed some useful interaction to help re-establish some hospitals.

At no stage in the early months of the operation was there any question of working jointly on what could have become a concerted overall plan for recovery. It should be realized that UNTAC coordination with the traditional UN agencies (WHO, UNICEF, etc.) was no better than it was with the NGOs. Yet there was a potentially very useful vehicle for this purpose: the monthly meeting of the coordination committee in the Ministry of Health. That was where all the aid organizations could meet, once a month, to explain their new projects and outline the most pressing problems facing the health system. The UNTAC representative only ever arrived very late, and then only as an observer. The need for neutrality was always invoked as an excuse for avoiding any active role at these meetings, held solely at the behest of the ruling political party. But UNTAC never proposed any alternative, nor did it delegate the coordination function to anyone else – and, worst of all, it never released the funds that would have been needed to make coordination more effective.

The UNHCR stands out as an honourable exception in this operation and an excellent example of efficiency and coordination. Its staff had the responsibility for repatriating the 385,000 Khmer refugees from the camps on the border of Thailand and it distinguished itself from the outset by its understanding of the situation and its willingness to work with the NGOs. This is probably largely due to the fact that the UNHCR knew the area so well, having worked for over ten years on the Thai–Cambodian frontier. Its strategy was different from the start: given the sparse funds available, it decided to distribute them effectively in several 'QUIPS' (Quick Impact Projects) to the NGOs and Red Cross teams which were often in place before the return of the refugees. They managed to defend the interests of their refugees without forgetting the general problems of the population, and were thus able to revive several existing hospitals and dispensaries for the joint benefit of all, both refugees and residents. They also succeeded in combining a repatriation operation with the beginnings of a genuine relaunching of the national health-care system.

CHALLENGES FOR THE FUTURE

Many countries throughout the world today are emerging deeply disturbed from the gigantic post-Cold War upheavals. While there are many opportunities for the international community to assist them in rebuilding, it is important to remember that the health sector has symbolic status for the populations involved. The rebuilding of health-care systems provides incomparable opportunities for contact with a country's people and structures. By making the most of the social dynamism which marks these periods of change, it provides effective leverage for the impetus to rebuild. At the same time, the revival of health systems calls for real political commitment which goes deeper than simple appearances because it is ultimately part of the foundation of social order.

Essential questions must be tackled, such as the formulation of a national health-care policy, the number and allocation of staff and the way the system is funded. In other words a superficial approach, both in theory and in practical action taken, is doomed to lead to failure and wastage. In this regard, the phase of situation assessment is a vital one. This phase is an essential precondition for all rebuilding operations; it provides the best guarantee of cohesion of the operation and a way of limiting the potential damage of technocratic arbitrariness.

Large-scale operations such as that of UNTAC in Cambodia do not have an automatic remit for reconstruction. However, as authority is concentrated in their hands in this critical period they must take better account of the context and the schemes under way, and must favour in particular those activities which will help to consolidate their own operations. In the health field it is essential to make use of the specialized agencies of the United Nations, the international agencies and NGOs which have the technical competence and credibility to provide help and undertake more focused activities. From the outset one must strive for effective sectoral coordination backed up by adequate financial resources. So it is vital to recognize and work together with the main players already present in the field. For all these reasons this necessary coordination should be carried out not by the special operation itself but by a specialized agency of the United Nations which is familiar with the problems of rebuilding health-care systems and resettling displaced people.

The purpose of funding must be, over and above the immediate objective of visibility, to provide the resources necessary for the long-term viability of projects. Assessment of the reconstruction programmes under way is an item most often singularly absent from the budget, yet reassessments of needs must be carried out regularly in order to decide in time on necessary adjustments and reorientation. In the absence of a universally valid model, and given the great diversity of possible situations, regular objective and independent evaluation is an essential aid in organizing reconstruction projects.

Philippe Biberson and Eric Goemaere

15

WHEN SUFFERING MAKES A GOOD STORY

Why did the Armenian earthquake in December 1988 mobilize the media and the public to such a degree when, in the same year, more than 250,000 people had died a lingering death as a result of famine and war in the Sudan? How could the extraordinary masquerade of the 'Romanian revolution', with its non-existent charnel-houses, its imaginary Libyan militia, its fake genocide, its humanitarian posturing and its pretend democrats, be played out right under our noses?

Why did the first film of the 1984 famine in Ethiopia fail to send more than a slight shiver down the spine of the United Kingdom while the second, broadcast three months later, galvanized the entire Western world into action? For what earthly reason did Liberia hit the headlines for several weeks in 1990 only to disappear without trace, despite the continuing war and the presence of a peacekeeping force?

Why are the bloody wars raging in Georgia and Nagorno-Karabakh in the Caucasus and in Tajikistan and Afghanistan in Central Asia given such short shrift, while our humanitarian incursions into Bosnia and Somalia are never off our TV screens?

And why, last but not least, was Somalia largely ignored by the media until August 1992 when, like Ethiopia seven years earlier, it suddenly became the centre of Western humanitarian attention and a testing-ground for a new brand of military intervention?

Members of humanitarian organizations, subject like anyone else to the fluctuating moods and whims of their societies, are by the very nature of their task constantly faced with these problems —not only because they need the material and moral support of the public if they are to act freely and effectively, but also because the reactions of governments and the United Nations to major crises are inextricably bound up with public opinion, whether they try to keep pace with it or manipulate it to obtain its support. In practice, these two processes often go hand in hand, with synchronization following on from manipulation. Lastly, over and above any international reaction, silence always feeds oppression: although knowing about a crisis does not solve it, the knowledge does at least pave the way for the most basic act of justice: if the guilty cannot be punished, at least the victims can be recognized.

There is, however, no universal law governing the process whereby an internal upheaval becomes an international event and then, perhaps, a crisis to which the international community is called upon to react. To realize this one has only to reflect that such a development depends on phenomena and interactions as complex as the collective psyche, the extent to which a society is prepared to take notice of issues foreign to its immediate concerns, the impact of the media, political decision-making processes and so forth.

HOW TO ENGINEER AN INTERNATIONAL EVENT

Our intention here is to provide food for thought, not answers. Our experience has led us to identify some of the ingredients – necessary, but not yet sufficient – needed to turn an upheaval into an international event:

1 Pictures, not words, turn an incident into an event, provided nowadays that they are available as a continuous flow to be tapped several times a day for cumulative effect – the only way to avoid being drowned by the flood of extraneous information. This alone is where the financial resources and editorial decisions of the newspapers come into play.
2 The upheaval must be isolated if it is not to be ousted once and for all by a parallel conflict: a television news service cannot cover two famines at once. The conflict in former Yugoslavia, given simultaneous coverage with Somalia, is a notable exception to this rule, doubtless because of its geographical position and its political implications.
3 There must be a mediator – a personality or a volunteer from a humanitarian organization – to 'authenticate' the victim, channel the emotion generated and provide both distance and a link between the spectator and the victim.
4 As well as the scene-setting, there must be a victim who is spontaneously acceptable in her or his own right to Western viewers: the Iraqi Shi'ites stand no more chance of passing this test than do the Palestinians in Kuwait or the Iranians, regardless of the hardship they may be suffering.

This set of rules governs the way in which news is fabricated, not the awareness process at work in a society. It works only if it can shake off the televisual consciousness of the world, which is often mistaken for knowledge. This technological optimism, which equates knowledge with conscience, is actually based on the 'global village' concept. Electronic news-gathering and rapid data transmission can be said to have reduced the world to the size of a village in which we are all neighbours. No one in an industrialized country today can claim not to know what is happening around them, since every house and every street in the global village is constantly washed by electronic waves broadcasting events as they happen. 'Give us 18 minutes and we will give you the universe' was the claim of the Satellite News Channel the day after Leonid Brezhnev's death. The Americans, along with all those with access to an unrestricted information source, actually heard about the death of the First Secretary to the Communist Party before the Soviets did. Since then satellites and the constant advances in perfecting and miniaturizing broadcasting and reception techniques have multiplied the effects of the technological achievement of which Satellite News Channel was so proud: no state can now claim a monopoly on information, and a tyrant's subjects learn of his death at the same time as the rest of the world.

The student revolt in Peking, the siege of Sarajevo, the Marine landings in Somalia and the riots in Los Angeles are served up to us every day at mealtimes, giving credence to the idea of a universal telepresence in which time and distance no longer exist. This divine quality of ubiquity turns the McLuhan galaxy into a kind of electronic Olympus, with a control room from which we newly-created gods can watch a world whose every tremor is scrutinized in real time and whose upheavals are instantly on our screens, producing a world conscience *ipso facto*. Everyone has access today to a vast fund of information on the chaotic progress of the world; every important event is at least signalled, even if it is engulfed immediately afterwards in the flood of information constantly on offer. No famine, no war, no oppressive regime has been totally and persistently neglected; hence the notion that horror is a thing of the past, since pictures are the worst enemy of indifference and arbitrary decisions – the pillar of the world conscience.

This technological optimism, which equates knowledge with conscience, is actually based on the symbolic show of strength (Bourdieu) which is the very recipe for the global village. This parable, invented by Marshall McLuhan when television was in its infancy, was quickly accepted as truth and gave rise to questions in which universal neighbourhood is taken for granted. There are, in fact, few things more questionable than this idea – an electronic version of the kingdom of Utopia – which is surely fired by the hope it brings and the strength of the headline it contains. The old adage of the man and the dog – 'dog bites man' is not news; 'man bites dog' is news – is often quoted as evidence that information is synonymous with the unexpected: trains arriving on time are never newsworthy, but may find a niche in advertising or propaganda. Where international news is concerned, though, the old adage is incomplete and misleading. Each person in a collectivity assimilates the necessarily elliptical language of information into the set of feelings, impressions and experiences which make up his or her specific context – into the idea she or he happens to have of the way dogs and men usually behave, i.e., the awareness that assaults by men on dogs are relatively rare. We have, in other words, a syntax in the sense of a set of rules governing the ways in which words or impressions are grouped, their levels of meaning and the common significance of the messages reaching us from our surroundings. The image of the emaciated Somali child gnawing at a root, its eyelids covered with flies, against a background of food convoys being pillaged, a scene we have watched a thousand times over, delivers a message whose primary meaning – a child in distress – is clear. The secondary meanings fit no ordinary syntax, belonging instead to a default system built up of earlier impressions: cracked, dried-out earth, criminal warlords, tribal warfare, population explosions, swarming illiterate masses, deadly epidemics – in short, a neo-mediaeval epic of misery. Such a scenario leaves no room for what really goes on in the society concerned – its various social structures, its power networks and hierarchies, its ideas and its culture. The only familiar landmark in this merciless, anachronistic landscape is the image of the victim. We shall return to this central point.

The Vietnam War demonstrated the power of the picture – its ability to mobilize public reserves of indignation at a time when the hoped-for political solutions had not yet been discredited. The flag of liberty that General Westmoreland wished to raise over the villages he had just napalmed was shot to pieces by the films and photographs taken by the journalists. Yet the opponents of this empire-building war were not interested in the methods by which the US militia conducted its operations. What they wanted was confirmation that their positions were justified, and that was provided by the photographs epitomizing the conflict: the terror of a small, naked girl running from a burning village and a South Vietnamese officer gunning down a Viet

Cong soldier in cold blood. These images did more than reveal hidden truths: they ratified an existing argument.

GOLDEN AGE FOR HUMANITARIANISM AND DARK DAYS FOR IDEOLOGY

Since the Vietnam War, no media tremor has succeeded in producing any perceptible display of, or change in, public opinion in the industrialized nations. Whether this is a fact to be rejoiced in or deplored, it remains true that only in the humanitarian field has society really expressed itself. From Uganda to Bosnia, Ethiopia to Armenia, Cambodia to Afghanistan, for better or for worse it is the humanitarian ethos that now prevails, with no other perspective in sight. At the same time, the power of television has become so great that it is now the focal point for the news. Since the early 1980s, headlines in the press have largely reflected those of the television news, and the latter now shoulders the heavy responsibility for deciding what is, and what is not 'news' – in effect, for creating the news.

These new changes took place independently of each other, but simultaneously. That coincidence was crucial to the years which followed, for it was during those years that humanitarianism really took off, seemingly the only form of public commitment still capable of being defended, occupying the territory vacated by hardline ideology and feeding on its very decline.

It was with the flight of refugees from South-East Asia, particularly the boat people of 1979, and the 1980 famine in Karamoja (Uganda) that we saw the first major televised humanitarian campaigns, resulting ultimately in the first ever military/humanitarian operations with the deployment of troops and their logistic support.

But communism, although widely perceived as intellectually moribund, was still alive and kicking as a political system, and East–West tensions limited operations of this type to a few insignificant territories. This was nevertheless the moment when the fate of mankind around the world began to form part of the daily lives of Westerners, vicariously through humanitarian aid.

The age of the 'French doctors' rapidly replaced that of heroes in the mould of Che Guevara – the latter more romantic, undoubtedly, but disqualified by reason of their enthusiasm for gulags. The humanitarian volunteer, a new, newsworthy figure, neither statesman nor guerrilla, but half-amateur and half-expert, began to appear at the flashpoints which light up the progress of history. Both actor and narrator, he has taken over where politics stopped, playing the front man with a sense of reality which he can reduce to a common denominator – the victim and the treatment he will be receiving – which immediately upstages any other social imagery expressed in the same terms.

Being a mixture of vehement protest, emergency medicine and sheer physical effort, this new form of humanitarian action seems to be ideal television news material. After all, its three components appeal immediately to the emotions. Quick, simple, and yielding immediately-visible results (at least in comparison with the political treatment of exotic problems), humanitarian action has the knack of showing itself in a form which is easy to understand and appreciate: the victim and his rescuer have become one of the totems of our age.

Man, as Marx observed, only ever sets himself problems he is capable of resolving: television news only ever brings us emotional images we are capable of sublimating. What this means in practice is that subjects virtually select themselves by a two-stage process. First, the physical timing imposed by the length and pace of the broadcast, which rule out the presentation of more than two international crises per news bulletin. Second, the symbolic status of 'victim', which can in effect only be granted in cases of unjustified or innocent suffering. It matters little whether the subject is the victim of mother nature's cruelty, of a senseless war (other peoples' wars are always senseless), of ruthless armed gangs, or of an evil tyrant —the point is that he must be 100 per cent victim, a non-participant. This means that the humanitarian doctor is almost in a position of having to apologize, to justify his actions, when caught in the act of giving treatment, in accordance with humanitarian principles, to combatants.

The high point in this lunatic requirement for purity of victim status was provided by the two great communicators of the 1980s, Presidents Ronald Reagan and Mikhail Gorbachev, with the rescue of two ice-trapped whales off the coast of Canada in October 1988. Little attention has been drawn to the significance of this spectacular farce's success. It was the prototype for other rococo events, an object lesson in the unexpected capacity of an emotionally-charged scenario to anaesthetize the critical faculties of the population at large. Here we had a hostile environment in the polar ice, innocent victims in the whales, a spectacular rescue with the giant helicopters and the blessing of authority in the persons of Messrs Reagan and Gorbachev, no less. Whilst all this was going on, and the front pages of the world's press were acclaiming the 'rescue of the century', in southern Sudan an organized famine was killing Dinkas by tens of thousands, in the silence of general indifference.

It can be noted in passing that the victims of a tyrant only become 'victims' when the tyrant has been perceived and labelled as such by western governments. Saddam Hussein became a fully-accredited producer of victims only when he overstepped the line which separates political friends from enemies. His gassing of 5,000 Kurds in 1988, and the repression they had suffered for years before, were irrelevant to his change of status. Armenia aroused the world's compassion in 1988 after the earthquake, but the same country's involvement in the war in Nagorno-Karabakh seems to have produced no victims worthy of interest. That is because their status is confused by their responsibility for the conflict. It is difficult to imagine Presidents Reagan and Gorbachev hastening to the rescue of a shoal of sharks or a pack of jackals.

The Gulf crisis provided an admirable showcase for the strength of the image perceived as truth, and the hijacking of emotion as a form of knowledge. Shortly before the United States Congress voted, a television report shook the nation: a girl (whose identity could not, for fear of reprisals, be revealed) sobbing as she reported the atrocities committed by the Iraqi soldiers as they invaded Kuwait City. She described the sacking of the hospitals' paediatric departments, the destruction of incubators, the infants left on the floor to die. Three hundred and nineteen premature infants had been killed in this way, we were told. This footage went around the world, inflaming opinion against the monstrous Iraqi baby-killer. This massacre of the innocents could not go unpunished: Congress, previously divided over Desert Storm, finally approved the operation by a majority of five. The rest is history.

And why not, after all? Well, simply because the interview was a fake: the interviewee was none other than the daughter of the Kuwaiti ambassador in Washington, playing with talent an imaginary role. One of America's leading communications agencies, financed by Kuwait, was behind this charade, less well-known than the Timisoara scam, but far more subtle. To depict accurately the outlines of your victim, you must first do the same for his oppressor, and Saddam Hussein's profile at the hands of his former protectors was that of the baby-devouring ogre of our fairy-tale nightmares. Two years earlier a Médecins Sans Frontières mission to the Kurdish villages gassed on Saddam's orders had had little press coverage despite the images it brought back; at the time, he had been a friend to the West, the rampart containing fundamentalist Islam within Iran. A neatly-assembled fabrication in a more receptive climate was able to outclass the reality of earlier massacres and oppression which at the time had been consigned to the international briefs in the inside pages.

THE OPPRESSOR, THE VICTIM AND THE GOOD SAMARITAN

For years, the civil war and the famine in Somalia belonged to this class of news in brief, sandwiched fleetingly between the birth of quintuplets in Australia and a railway crash in India. The human drama triggered by this political upheaval became properly visible only when political personalities began to show interest. Events in Somalia required strong words from the Secretary-General of the United Nations, and visits by US Senator Nancy Kasselbaum and the French Minister for Humanitarian Action, Dr Bernard Kouchner, before the tragedy became news, when the famine had already reached and passed its peak after months of deepening crisis. It was at that point that Somalia burst onto the West's consciousness, in images of dying children and armed gangs roaming a wilderness.

Once the victims have been identified as *bona fide* by acknowledged mediators, they can become the object of our compassion, and their oppressors that of our opprobrium. Thus by August 1992 the scene had been set, the four criteria had been met, and Act One could begin, with the United Nations' laborious relief deployment. With Act Two came a brutal heightening in the dramatic intensity of events, as the Secretary-General's special envoy resigned. In late November the figure of 80 per cent of food aid failing to reach the right people began to emerge, and the Secretary-General himself took this figure up, although it had no known factual basis, and a fortnight earlier, all those actually involved estimated the losses at 30–40 per cent of the total.

Widely acclaimed – except by those actually present in Somalia, the NGOs – as a self-evident truth, this 'news' promoted events to the rank of crisis, opening the possibility of a military humanitarian aid operation. Thus was the way opened for Act Three: Ambassador Sahnoun, the diplomat attempting to renew the political dialogue, was replaced by a military command with the task of neutralizing the armed gangs and warlords responsible for the famine. This spectacle would reach its high point on 8 December with the landing of the US Marines on the beaches of Mogadishu. The humanitarian teams, unable to recognize themselves or their mission in the euphoria of the moment, saw these events as harbingers of trouble; their premonitions proved all too well-founded.

No doubt the origins of this escalation lay in the confusion which followed the Gulf War and the impotence of the international community faced with the Bosnian war of ethnic cleansing, alongside other political issues. No doubt the total breakdown of state structures and the level of violence attained required a firm reaction. But the fact is that the lack of direction we are now witnessing in Somalia results from applying the same mental processes as were applied in the campaign for baby seals massacred by ruthless hunters on deserted ice-floes. And that the problems faced by this operation result largely from the return of a political reality which this simplistic, reassuring imagery was incapable of turning around.

Men, as Machiavelli observed, judge by what they see. What becomes of their judgement when the eye is replaced by the telephoto lens, and a point of view is replaced by a camera-angle? Somalia provides the answer: the map is taken to be the ground, and the image is taken to be reality. Even the sound-bite can be taken for image: the principal effect of the statements by General Philippe Morillon, head of the UNPROFOR in Bosnia, on the establishment of 'safe areas' was to popularize the expression 'safe areas' and, by a slight shift in emphasis, imply that such areas actually existed, and that the Bosnians were therefore safe. A high-profile operation in Srebrenica and a close-up of a few Blue Helmets was all that was then needed: through the telescope of the television news, Srebrenica became the whole of Bosnia, and one instant of success wiped out the accumulated deficit of failure.

HUMANITARIAN ACTION ON THE BRIDGE BETWEEN INFORMATION AND COMMUNICATION

Government, as Hobbes pointed out as long ago as the seventeenth century, is a matter of belief. Hobbes is all the more relevant in this age of the cathodic rite – the first in history, Régis Debray tells us, in which men actually believe the evidence of their eyes. Much of the blame for this lies with the fact that the entertainment and communications industry (which the television companies effectively are) has a powerful hold over the news. But it would be absurd to hold journalists or media organizations solely responsible for the over-simplifications and the abusively emotional presentation of complex situations: presentation, selection and subjectivity are an inevitable part of journalism: that job cannot be reduced to simply recording fact. Austerity is no guarantee of truth, and the dream of worldwide transparency is no more than a totalitarian nightmare.

What we face here is a problem in society: compassion, otherwise known as solidarity, is tending to degenerate into pity, when it should be growing into calls for justice. Information, frequently distressing, is subtly replaced by 'communication', which is always middle-of-the-road. The 'satisfaction index' and the 'press book' are deemed to express the results, and the display of virtuous intentions and humanitarian oratory have become substitutes for policy.

This situation may be short-term, but even without it, it is difficult to imagine that the West will stop choosing its 'victims' on the basis of whim and interest. Journalists certainly have a responsibility to consider the consequences of their professional practices, but the humanitarian organizations also have two responsibilities no less great. First, they must continue to exploit in the best interests of the victim the potential offered by the popular media. Second, they must consider their own professional practices, and demonstrate that what they are doing is founded on principles more solidly based, and hence more demanding, than the appeals to the emotions which are so tempting to exploit. That is the price which will have to be paid, if the true ethos implicit in humanitarian organizations is to be distinguished from the unfeeling morality which is beginning to mark them. That, in particular, is the price which will have to be paid if humanitarian aid is to retain its respect for the individuals it seeks to help. That is the price which will have to be paid if the ethics implicit in humanitarian organizations are to survive in the world of the media, and neither give up nor resort to demagogy.

Rony Brauman

MSF WORLDWIDE

Operational sections

Belgium
Médecins Sans Frontières
Artsen zonder Grenzen
Rue Deschampheleer 24
B–1080 Brussels
Tel.   32–2–414.03.00
Fax   32–2–411.82.60

France
Médecins Sans Frontières
8 rue Saint Sabin
F–75011 Paris
Tel.   33–1.40.21.29.29
Fax   33–1.48.06.68.68

Holland
Artsen zonder Grenzen
Max Euweplein 40
NL–1017 MD Amsterdam
Tel.   31–20.52.08.700
Fax   31–20.620.51.70/72

Luxembourg
Médecins Sans Frontières
70 Route de Luxembourg
L–7240 Bereldange
Tel.   352–33.25.15
Fax   352–33.51.33

Spain
Medicos Sin Fronteras
Avda Portal del Angel N°1, 1
E–08002 Barcelona
Tel.   34–3–412.52.52
Fax   34–3–302.28.89

Switzerland
Médecins Sans Frontières
1 Clos de la Fonderie
CH–1227 Carouge
Tel.   41/22.300.44.45
Fax   41/22.300.44.14

Branch offices

Australia
24 Angus Avenue
Epping NSW 2121
Tel.   61/2/482.15.00
Fax   61/2/875.22.88.

Canada
56 The Esplanade, Suite 202
Toronto, Ontario M5E 1A7
Tel.   1/416/366.67.02
      or   863.67.33

Denmark
Strandvejen 171,1
DK–2900 Hellerup
Tel.   45/31/62.63.01
Fax   45/39/40.14.92

Germany
Adenauer Allee 50
D–53113 Bonn
Tel.   49/228/22.97.93
Fax   49/228/22.03.71

*Greece**
Médecins Sans Frontières
11 Rue Paioniou
GR–10440 Athens
Tel.   30/1/88.35.334
      or   88.35.665
Fax   30/1/882.99.88

Italy
Via Ostiense 6/E
I–00152 Roma
Tel.   39/6/57.300.900/901
Fax   39/6/57.300.902

Japan
Honda Building 4F
2–14–5 Takadanobaba
Shinjuku-Ku Tokyo 169
Tel.   81/3/52.72.18.41
Fax   81/3/52.72.88.60

* in the process of being set up as a section

Sweden
Vulcanusgatan 8
S–113 21 Stockholm
Tel.   46/8/31.02.17
Fax   46/8/31.42.90

UK
3–4 St Andrews Hill
London EC4V 5BY
Tel.   44/71/329.69.39
Fax   44/71/329.69.36

USA
30 Rockefeller Plaza
Suite 5425
NY 10112, New York
Tel.   1/212/649.59.61
Fax   1/212/246.58.44
        or   246.85.77

UN Liaison Office Geneva
14b rue des Cordiers
CH-1207 Geneva
Tel.   41/22/786.47.19
Fax   41/22/786.47.05

Intl. Office
Boulevard Leopold II 209
B–1080 Brussels
Tel.   32/2/426.55.52
Fax   32/2/426.75.35